MORE 4U!

the clinics

This Clinics series is available online.

Here's what you get:

- Full text of EVERY issue from 2002 to NOW
- Figures, tables, drawings, references and more
- Searchable: find what you need fast

Search | All Clinics ▼ | for | | GO

- Linked to MEDLINE and Elsevier journals
- E-alerts

INDIVIDUAL SUBSCRIBERS

Click **Register** and follow instructions

You'll need an account number

LOG ON TODAY. IT'S FAST AND EASY.

Your subscriber account number is on your mailing label →

This is your copy of:
THE CLINICS OF NORTH AMERICA
CXXX **2296532-2** 2 Mar 05
J.H. DOE, MD
531 MAIN STREET
CENTER CITY, NY 10001-001

BOUGHT A SINGLE ISSUE? Sorry, you won't be able to access full text online. Please subscribe today to get complete content by contacting customer service at 800 645 2552 (US and Canada) or 407 345 4000 (outside US and Canada) or via email at elsols@elsevier.com.

NEW!

Now also available for INSTITUTIONS

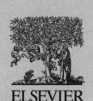

ELSEVIER

Works/Integrates with MD Consult

Available in a variety of packages: Collections containing 14, 31 or 50 Clinics titles

Or Collection upgrade for existing MD Consult customers

Call today! 877-857-1047 or e-mail: mdc.groupinfo@elsevier.com

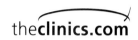

RADIOLOGIC CLINICS
of North America

Hepatic Imaging

RICHARD C. SEMELKA, MD
Guest Editor

September 2005 • Volume 43 • Number 5

SAUNDERS

An Imprint of Elsevier, Inc.
PHILADELPHIA   LONDON   TORONTO   MONTREAL   SYDNEY   TOKYO

W.B. SAUNDERS COMPANY
A Division of Elsevier Inc.

1600 John F. Kennedy Boulevard • Suite 1800 • Philadelphia, Pennsylvania 19103-2899

http://www.theclinics.com

RADIOLOGIC CLINICS OF NORTH AMERICA
September 2005
Editor: Barton Dudlick

Volume 43, Number 5
ISSN 0033-8389
ISBN 1-4160-2762-9

Radiologic Clinics of North America (ISSN 0033-8389) is published bimonthly by W.B. Saunders Company. Corporate and editorial offices: 1600 John F. Kennedy Boulevard, Suite 1800, Philadelphia, Pennsylvania 19103-2899. Accounting and circulation offices: 6277 Sea Harbor Drive, Orlando, FL 32887-4800. Periodicals postage paid at Orlando, FL 32862, and additional mailing offices. Subscription prices are USD 220 per year for US individuals, USD 331 per year for US institutions, USD 110 per year for US students and residents, USD 255 per year for Canadian individuals, USD 405 per year for Canadian institutions, USD 299 per year for international individuals, USD 405 per year for international institutions and USD 150 per year for Canadian and foreign students/residents. To receive student and resident rate, orders must be accompanied by name of affiliated institution, date of term, and the *signature* of program/residency coordinator on institution letterhead. Orders will be billed at individual rate until proof of status is received. Foreign air speed delivery is included in all *Clinics* subscription prices. All prices are subject to change without notice. POSTMASTER: Send address changes to *Radiologic Clinics of North America*, W.B. Saunders Company, Periodicals Fulfillment, Orlando, FL 32887-4800. **Customer Service: 800-654-2452 (US). From outside of the US, call (+1) 407-345-4000.**

Radiologic Clinics of North America also is published in Greek by Paschalidis Medical Publications, Athens, Greece.

Radiologic Clinics of North America is covered in *Index Medicus, EMBASE/Excerpta Medica, Current Contents/Life Sciences, Current Contents/Clinical Medicine, RSNA Index to Imaging Literature, BIOSIS, Science Citation Index,* and *ISI/BIOMED.*

Printed in the United States of America.

GOAL STATEMENT

The goal of the *Radiologic Clinics of North America* is to keep practicing radiologists and radiology residents up to date with current clinical practice in radiology by providing timely articles reviewing the state of the art in patient care.

ACCREDITATION

The *Radiologic Clinics of North America* is planned and implemented in accordance with the Essential Areas and Policies of the Accreditation Council for Continuing Medical Education (ACCME) through the joint sponsorship of the University of Virginia School of Medicine and Elsevier. The University of Virginia School of Medicine is accredited by the ACCME to provide continuing medical education for physicians.

The University of Virginia School of Medicine designates this educational activity for a maximum of 90 category 1 credits per year, 15 category 1 credits per issue, toward the AMA Physician's Recognition Award. Each physician should claim only those credits that he/she actually spent in the activity.

The American Medical Association has determined that physicians not licensed in the US who participate in this CME activity are eligible for AMA PRA category 1 credit.

AMA PRA category 1 credit can be earned by reading the text material, taking the examination online at http://www. theclinics.com/home/cme, and completing the evaluation. After taking the test, your will be required to review any and all incorrect answers. Following completion of the test and the evaluation, your credit will be awarded and you may print your certificate.

FACULTY DISCLOSURE

As a provider accredited by the Accreditation Council for Continuing Medical Education (ACCME), the Office of Continuing Medical Education of the University of Virginia School of Medicine must ensure balance, independence, objectivity, and scientific rigor in all its individually sponsored or jointly sponsored educational activities. All authors/editors participating in a sponsored activity are expected to disclose to the readers any significant financial interest or other relationship (1) with the manufacturer(s) of any commercial product(s) and/or provider(s) of commercial services discussed in an educational presentation and (2) with any commercial supporters of the activity (significant financial interest or other relationship can include such things as grants or research support, employee, consultant, stock holder, member of speakers bureau, etc.) The intent of this disclosure is not to prevent authors/editors with a significant financial or other relationship from writing an article, but rather to provide readers with information on which they can make their own judgments. It remains for the readers to determine whether the author's/editor's interest or relationships may influence the article with regard to exposition or conclusion.

The authors/editors listed below have identified no professional or financial affiliations related to their article:
N. Cem Balci, MD; Larissa Braga, MD, PhD; Charles Burke, MD; Raman Danrad, MD; Barton Dudlick, Acquisitions Editor; Ulrich Guller, MD, MHSc; Shahid M. Hussain, MD; Amir H. Khandani, MD, PhD; Yuko Kono, MD, PhD; Diego R. Martin, MD, PhD; Robert F. Mattrey, MD; Aytekin Oto, MD; Richard C. Semelka, MD; Janio Szklaruk, MD, PhD; Eric P. Tamm, MD; and, Susan M. Weeks, MD.

The author listed below has identified the following professional or financial affiliations related to his article:
Richard L. Wahl, MD has received research grant support and honoraria from GE Medical, and honoraria from Philips and Cardinal Health.

Disclosure of discussion of non-FDA approved uses for pharmaceutical products and/or medical devices:
The University of Virginia School of Medicine, as an ACCME provider, requires that all authors/editors identify and disclose any "off label" uses for pharmaceutical products and/or for medical devices. The University of Virginia School of Medicine recommends that each reader fully review all the available data on new products or procedures prior to instituting them with patients.

All authors/editors who provided disclosures will not be discussing any off-label uses except:
Yuko Kono, MD, PhD and Robert F. Mattrey, MD discuss the use of ultrasound contrast agents in liver imaging. The use of ultrasound contrast agents in liver imaging is off label for any agents (not specified) approved in the US.

TO ENROLL

To enroll in the Radiologic Clinics of North America Continuing Medical Education program, call customer service at 1-800-654-2452 or sign up online at http://www.theclinics.com/home/cme. The CME program is available to subscribers for an additional annual fee of USD 195.

FORTHCOMING ISSUES

RECENT ISSUES

GUEST EDITOR

RICHARD C. SEMELKA, MD, Professor (Radiology); Director, MR Services; and Vice Chair, Clinical Research, Department of Radiology, School of Medicine, University of North Carolina at Chapel Hill, North Carolina

CONTRIBUTORS

N. CEM BALCI, MD, Associate Professor (Radiology), Department of Radiology, Saint Louis University, St. Louis, Missouri

LARISSA BRAGA, MD, PhD, Research Fellow, Department of Radiology, School of Medicine, University of North Carolina at Chapel Hill, Chapel Hill, North Carolina

CHARLES BURKE, MD, Assistant Professor, Department of Radiology, School of Medicine, University of North Carolina at Chapel Hill, Chapel Hill, North Carolina

RAMAN DANRAD, MD, Fellow, Abdominal Imaging, Department of Radiology, Emory University School of Medicine, Atlanta, Georgia

ULRICH GULLER, MD, MHSc, Surgical Resident, Divisions of General Surgery and Surgical Research, Department of Surgery, University of Basel, Basel, Switzerland

SHAHID M. HUSSAIN, MD, Head, Section of Abdominal Imaging, Department of Radiology, Erasmus MC, Rotterdam, The Netherlands

AMIR H. KHANDANI, MD, PhD, Assistant Professor (Radiology); and Director, PET Imaging, Section of Nuclear Medicine, Department of Radiology, University of North Carolina, Chapel Hill, North Carolina

YUKO KONO, MD, PhD, Assistant Research Scientist, Department of Radiology, University of California at San Diego, San Diego, California

DIEGO R. MARTIN, MD, PhD, Professor; and Director, Magnetic Resonance Imaging, Department of Radiology, Emory University School of Medicine, Atlanta, Georgia

ROBERT F. MATTREY, MD, Professor, Department of Radiology, University of California at San Diego, San Diego, California

AYTEKIN OTO, MD, Associate Professor (Radiology); and Director, Body Imaging, Department of Radiology, University of Texas Medical Branch at Galveston, Galveston, Texas

RICHARD C. SEMELKA, MD, Professor (Radiology); Director, MR Services; and Vice Chair, Clinical Research, Department of Radiology, School of Medicine, University of North Carolina at Chapel Hill, North Carolina

JANIO SZKLARUK, MD, PhD, Assistant Professor, Department of Diagnostic Radiology, MD Anderson Cancer Center, University of Texas, Houston, Texas

ERIC P. TAMM, MD, Assistant Professor, Department of Diagnostic Radiology, MD Anderson Cancer Center, University of Texas, Houston, Texas

RICHARD L. WAHL, MD, Henry N. Wagner Jr. MD Professor of Nuclear Medicine; Professor (Oncology); Director, Nuclear Medicine/PET; and Vice Chair, New Technology and Business Development, Russell H. Morgan Department of Radiology and Radiological Science, The Johns Hopkins University School of Medicine, Johns Hopkins Hospital, Baltimore, Maryland

SUSAN M. WEEKS, MD, Chief, Vascular and Interventional Radiology; and Associate Professor, Department of Radiology, School of Medicine, University of North Carolina at Chapel Hill, Chapel Hill, North Carolina

CONTRIBUTORS

CONTENTS

ELSEVIER
SAUNDERS

Radiol Clin N Am 43 (2005) xi

RADIOLOGIC
CLINICS
of North America

Preface

Hepatic Imaging

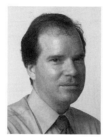

Richard C. Semelka, MD
Guest Editor

The liver is the most important organ in the abdomen, and the only one without which we cannot go on living. The greatest range of benign and malignant disease processes also afflict the liver. Because of the importance of the liver, and because it is one of the most common locales for spread of malignant disease, the liver is the abdominal organ of greatest interest for the use of imaging studies. As a result, much research and many developments for a variety of imaging modalities is geared toward improved visualization of liver disease. It is therefore appropriate that this issue of *Radiologic Clinics of North America* is devoted to hepatic imaging.

A number of authorities describe herein the developments and current clinical status of individual imaging technologies: ultrasound, CT, PET, and MR imaging. The range and behavior of contrast agents and mechanisms currently has the greatest spectrum and complexity with MR imaging, so this is described in its own article. Because of the common involvement of the liver by primary or secondary malignant disease, a number of local therapeutic interventional approaches have been developed, which is also described in its own article. Furthermore, malignant disease of the liver is no longer considered a terminal event, but rather a chronic disease state, and as more varied forms of treatment are developed and employed, it is becoming increasingly more common and important that evaluation of therapeutic response in the liver is performed accurately. This is also described in its own article. Finally to distill the myriad developments in the different imaging modalities and present an overview of a comparative evaluation of these modalities, a separate article has been devoted to analyzing their appropriate use in current clinical practice.

Richard C. Semelka, MD
Professor, Radiology
Director, MR Services
Vice Chair, Clinical Research
Department of Radiology
School of Medicine
University of North Carolina at Chapel Hill
2000 Old Clinic Building
Campus Box 7510
Chapel Hill, NC 27599-7510, USA
E-mail address: richsem@med.unc.edu

ELSEVIER
SAUNDERS

Radiol Clin N Am 43 (2005) 815 – 826

RADIOLOGIC
CLINICS
of North America

Ultrasound of the Liver

Yuko Kono, MD, PhD*, Robert F. Mattrey, MD

Department of Radiology, University of California at San Diego, 200 West Arbor Drive, San Diego, CA 92103–8756, USA

Ultrasound is widely accessible, relatively inexpensive, noninvasive, and portable; provides high spatial and temporal resolution; can be repeated frequently; and remains the first choice in many institutions for the screening of patients with suspected liver disease. For the screening of hepatocellular carcinoma (HCC) in high-risk patients with liver cirrhosis a combination of ultrasound and alpha fetoprotein every 6 months is recommended in most countries [1]. With recent advances in ultrasound including power Doppler imaging, tissue harmonic imaging, ultrasound contrast agents, and contrast-specific imaging, the clinical usefulness has increased dramatically, although limitations remain. The changes with the greatest impact on current imaging are the introduction of contrast agents and the adaptation of instruments to contrast-specific imaging. This article focuses on contrast imaging.

Ultrasound contrast agents

The first observation of ultrasound contrast was in 1968 when Gramiak and Shah [2] injected saline into the ascending aorta and observed better echo signals in the lumen of the aorta and heart chambers because of the production of microbubbles. Agitated saline was used for contrast echocardiography to delineate intracardiac shunts, to define congenital heart disease, and to examine the right-sided valves until commercial contrast agents started to develop in the 1980s. Although effective enhancement of the liver was

achieved with liquid emulsion [3] and solid particles [4], which reached clinical testing [5], it is the microbubble-based agents that have affected the clinical practice of ultrasound liver imaging. One of the reasons for the success of microbubbles is the ability to design instruments specifically to interact with and image these contrast agents permitting the use of miniscule doses [6]. Table 1 lists the commercial microbubble-based agents, their development status, and their properties. Because air microbubbles had an extremely short intravascular dwell-time, the first approach was to stabilize the bubbles. The first agent was Echovist (Schering AG, Berlin, Germany) in 1982, which enabled right side enhancement only, followed by Levovist in1985, which achieved enhancement of the left ventricle. Echovist and Levovist were approved in Europe, Japan, and Canada. Albunex (MBI, San Diego, California) was the first agent approved by the US Food and Drug Administration for United States distribution in 1994. Albunex is an air microbubble with an albumin shell. Both Albunex and Levovist use air as the gas. The use of low plasma soluble gas to increase the persistence of the microbubble was first introduced in the early 1990s. Optison (MBI) used perfluorocarbon gas with Albunex shell and was approved by the Food and Drug Administration for commercial use in 1997 for left ventricular opacification and endocardial border detection. Although most of the agents developed thereafter use perfluorocarbon gas with varying emulsifiers as shells, SonoVue (Bracco, Milan, Italy) uses sulfur hexafluoride. SonoVue is currently only approved in Europe. Definity (Bristol Myers Squibb, New York, New York) in 2001 and Imagent (IMCOR, San Diego, California) in 2002 are microbubbles with perfluorocarbon gas in a lipid

---

* Corresponding author.
E-mail address: ykono@ucsd.edu (Y. Kono).

Table 1
Echo contrast agents

Agent research name	Generic name	Company	Shell	Gas	Status
Levovist SHU 508A[a]	Galactose/palmitic acid	Schering AG	Galactose/palmitic acid	Air	EU-approved: LVO/doppler Canada-approved: LVO/doppler
Optison FS069[a]	Perfluetren protein microspheres	Amersham Health	Human serum albumin	Octafluoropropane	USA and EU approved: LVO/EBD/doppler Canada-approved: LVO/EBD Investigational: MCE
Definity DMP 115[a]	Perfluetren lipid microsphere suspension	Bristol-Myers Squibb Medical Imaging	Lipids: DPPA, DPPC, MPEG5000 DPPE	Octafluoropropane	USA-approved: LVO/EBD Canada-approved: LVO/EBD Investigational: MCE
Imagent AF0150[a]	Dimyristoylphatidylcholine/ perflexane	IMCOR Pharmaceuticals	Lipid: DMPC	Perfluorohexane/nitrogen	USA-approved: LVO/EBD Investigational: MCE
SonoVue BR1[a]	Sulphur hexafluoride	Bracco Diagnostics	Lipids: macrogol 4000, DSPC, DPPG, palmitic acid	Sulfurhexafluoride	EU-approved: LVO/EBD, micro- and macrovascular doppler (noncardiac) Investigational: MCE
Sonazoid NC100100	Decafluorobutane lipid	Amersham Health	Lipid stabilized (not disclosed)[b]	Perfluorobutane[b]	Development in USA and EU suspended[a]
BR14	Perfluorobutane	Bracco Diagnostics	Not disclosed	Perfluorobutane[c]	Investigational: MCE

Abbreviations: DMPC, dimyristoylphosphatidalcholine; DPPA, dipalmatoylphosphatidic acid; DPPC, dipalmatoylphosphatidylcholine MPEG5000; DPPE, dipalmatoylphosphatidalethanolamine; DPPG, dipalmitoylphosphatidylglycerol sodium; DSPC, distearoylphosphatidylcholine; EBD, endocardial border detection; EU, European Union; LVO, left ventricular opacification; MCE, myocardial contrast echocardiography.

  [a] *Data from* Approval documents: package inserts, summary basis for approval, product monographs, and news releases. 428 Ultrasound in Medicine and Biology, vol. 30, no. 4, 2004.

  [b] *Data from* Hvattum E, Normann PT, Oulie I, et al. Determination of perfluorobutane in rat blood by automatic headspace capillary gas chromatography and selected ion monitoring mass spectrometry. JPBA 2001;24:487–94.

  [c] *Data from* Seidel G, Meyer K, Algermissen C, Broillet A. Harmonic imaging of the brain parenchyma using a perfluorobutane-containing ultrasound contrast agent. Ultrasound in Med & Biol 2001;27:915–8.

Modified from Miller AP. Contrast echocardiography: new agents. Ultrasound Med Biol 2004;30:425–34 [Table 1].

shell that are also approved by the Food and Drug Administration for cardiology applications. No contrast agents are currently available for radiology applications in the United States [7].

Optison, Definity, Imagent, and SonoVue have slight differences in sensitivity and fragility to ultrasound, duration of enhancement, and so forth, but their overall performance is similar and they are all useful in many applications including liver tumor characterization [8–10]. Levovist is somewhat different from the other agents. It produces a weaker signal and is the only approved agent with liver-specific uptake other than transient mechanical trapping within the hepatic sinusoids [11]. Levovist has also been used in hepatic transit time analysis [12]. Sonazoid, like other perfluorocarbon-based agents, has a vascular phase but like Levovist also has specific liver uptake. Its development, however, is underway only in Japan and is currently suspended in the United States and Europe.

An important and common characteristic of all these agents is that they have nonlinear acoustic behavior and are easily destroyed by ultrasound. These characteristics are important to understand the principle of contrast-specific imaging techniques and low mechanical index (MI) and intermittent imaging.

Contrast-specific imaging technique

Microbubbles are effective ultrasound scatterers because of the large impedance difference between the surrounding fluid (eg, blood) and the encapsulated gas. Burns [13] has presented a detailed discussion on this topic. Some of the issues pertinent to liver imaging are detailed here. Because microbubbles, unlike tissues, resonate when exposed to ultrasound, they also become transmitters. The transmitted sound is at the same frequency as the sound that excited them if the applied sound pressure is low. At higher pressure, bubble expansion and contraction become nonlinear. The exposure of microbubbles to sound forces them to contract and expand their diameter several fold at their resonant frequency. In addition to the weakening and disruption of their protective shell, the gas body is fragmented into multiple smaller microbubbles resulting in their collapse and destruction. Bubble disruption and collapse generates a broadband frequency that includes the subharmonics and higher harmonics. Contrast-specific imaging takes advantage of these characteristics to manipulate image contrast. Harmonic imaging, which includes second harmonic B-mode imaging, harmonic color and power Doppler imag-

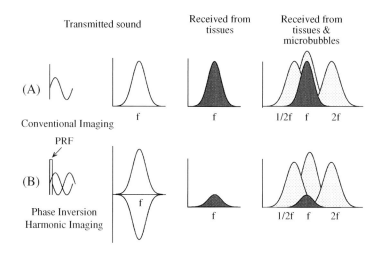

Fig. 1. Principle of phase inversion harmonic imaging. (*A*) Conventional ultrasound designed to image tissues. The fundamental frequency (*f*) is transmitted and received to generate images. The signal from microbubbles (contrast agents) contains different frequencies including fundamental (*f*), second harmonic (*2f*), and subharmonic (*2/f*) frequencies because of the nonlinear behavior of microbubbles (see Fig. 2). It is hard to discriminate the microbubble signal from tissue signals when only the fundamental frequency is used to generate images. (*B*) Phase inversion harmonic imaging transmits two consecutive pulses, one the opposite of the other. The signal from tissue is nearly canceled, but because of their nonlinear behavior the microbubble signal remains. The image generated by this technique consists mainly of nonlinear signals from microbubbles. This method is currently used worldwide to image ultrasound contrast agents.

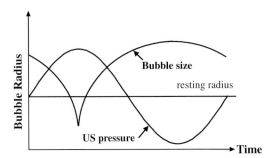

Fig. 2. Microbubble response in a sound field. Microbubbles shrink to a certain degree when the ultrasound pressure is positive but expand much more so when ultrasound pressure is negative. This nonlinear behavior in the sound field generates harmonic frequencies (see Fig. 1).

ing, and phase (pulse)-inversion technique, is a powerful sonographic contrast imaging technique. Among these contrast-specific techniques, the most important and currently widely used in liver imaging is phase (pulse)-inversion gray-scale imaging. A more detailed description of the various contrast-specific approaches is available [13].

Phase-inversion harmonic imaging transmits two ultrasound pulses and receives broadband signals, where the second pulse is inverted and slightly delayed relative to the first (Fig. 1). Tissue scatterers behave similarly during the positive and negative pressure phases of the pulse, and the reflections from the first and second pulses are equal and opposite and cancel each other. Bubbles behave differently during the positive and negative pressure phases of the pulse because they can expand several-fold at peak negative pressure with limited compression at peak positive pressure (Fig. 2) and result in stronger signal. Phase-inversion harmonic imaging is superior compared with second harmonic imaging that was developed first, because of its higher spatial resolution, more effective tissue suppression, and greater signal from microbubbles, and is currently used in most of the high-end ultrasound machines [6].

Low mechanical index and intermittent imaging

Microbubbles are easily destroyed by acoustic pressure. Low MI and intermittent imaging are two ways to image microbubbles to obtain sufficient contrast enhancement and extract physiologic data because CT and MR imaging dynamic series can be extracted. Low MI, real-time imaging provides an angiographic-like detail of the vasculature of an organ or tumor and the filling and enhancement of

tissues. Intermittent imaging performed at optimal MI produces higher-quality images, particularly in the far field, and with manipulation of the interval delay provides similar physiologic data as low MI imaging. After most of the ultrasound manufactures succeeded in obtaining good sensitivity to contrast with adequate spatial resolution with low MI imaging, however, the necessity for intermittent imaging declined. Because microbubble destruction invariably occurs, even at low MI, understanding the principles of intermittent imaging is important. As microbubbles in the imaging plane are destroyed with the imaging frame, the contrast on the following frame depends on the number of microbubbles that enter the plane between the two frames [14]. With short delay times image contrast reflects blood flow differences, whereas with long delay times image contrast reflects blood volume differences (Fig. 3). Hemangiomas show typical enhancement pattern of gradual filling with longer interval delay and high blood volume compared with surrounding liver when imaged with long interval delay with 10 to 15 seconds (Fig. 4).

Liver tumor characterization and detection

The gray-scale harmonic contrast-enhanced ultrasound has been used for liver tumor characterization and is proved to be very useful [15–17]. The characteristics of dynamic enhancement pattern of hepatic

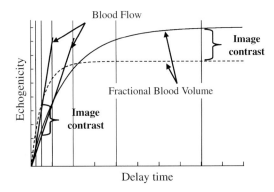

Fig. 3. Change in tissue signal and image contrast between two tissues with different blood flow and fractional blood volume as the inter-frame delay is increased. As microbubbles are destroyed by ultrasound pressure it is possible with intermittent imaging to assess blood flow and blood volume difference within the liver. With a shorter delay time, image contrast reflects blood flow differences, whereas with a longer delay time image contrast reflects fractional blood volume differences. This concept is important in liver tumor characterization.

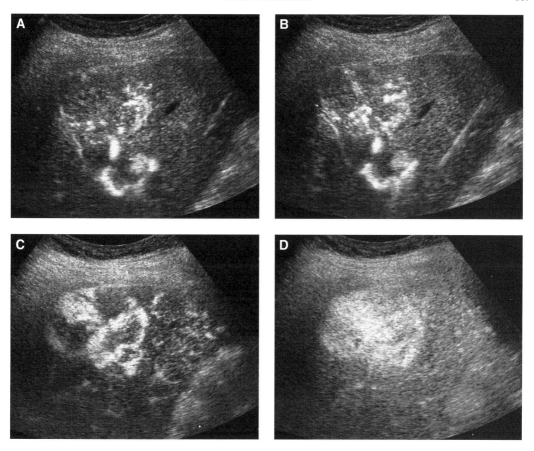

Fig. 4. Hemangioma with contrast-enhanced ultrasound shown in four phases of contrast filling. (*A* and *B*) Arterial- phase images show supply vessels with interrupted peripheral filling of the lesion. (*C*) At 1-second delay further filling of the tumor is noted, which is expansion of the puddles seen in (*B*). (*D*) With 5-second delay the lesion is nearly completely filled and the lesion has become more echogenic than liver consistent with its higher fractional blood volume.

tumors, such as HCC, metastatic liver tumors, hemangioma, focal nodular hyperplasia, and adenoma, are very similar to those with contrast-enhanced CT and MR imaging [18–20] despite of the fundamental difference from CT and MR imaging agents that microbubbles are pure intravascular agents.

Although Doppler signal is easily enhanced by contrast media, Doppler techniques are suboptimal for liver tumor imaging postcontrast because of blooming and flash artifacts, poor spatial resolution of color Doppler, and poor temporal resolution of power Doppler [21].

It is difficult to diagnose liver tumors with Doppler alone, which only provides detail of larger vessels and their anatomic relationship. Although it is sufficient to accept that a lesion is vascular by demonstrating the existence of Doppler signal within it, the difference between lesions and background tissue can be too subtle to aid in detection. Because most of the blood volume is in capillaries and flow in capillaries is very slow, Doppler techniques are severely handicapped. B-mode imaging makes no assumptions related to flow or motion. It strictly displays the location and intensity of the background signal. This characteristic places B-mode techniques at a significant advantage, because the received signal is influenced by microbubbles located in all tissue spaces including capillaries and wherever microbubbles are trapped. Analogous to CT, enhancement of the parenchyma to achieve a tissue blush may be the most sensitive technique to detect perfusion abnormalities. Further, gray-scale imaging has been optimized to maximize contrast, spatial, and temporal resolution that exceed those of color or power Doppler techniques.

The advantage of ultrasound dynamic enhancement compared with CT and MR imaging is that ultrasound dynamic enhancement is real-time imaging (10–20 frames per second) with greater spatial and contrast resolution to provide more detail. Focal nodular hyperplasia, for example, is probably best characterized with contrast-enhanced ultrasound because the central feeding artery and spoke wheel vessels are better seen because of the high spatial and temporal resolution (Fig. 5). Other examples of HCC and metastatic liver tumors with contrast enhancement are shown in Figs. 6 and 7. Table 2 shows typical enhancement patterns of hepatic tumors with contrast-enhanced ultrasound.

For differential diagnosis of hepatic tumors, intermittent imaging with various time delay, and real-time dynamic enhancement, is important. With long delay times when image contrast reflects fractional blood volume and allows the penetration of bubbles to the capillary level, improvements in lesion detection and margination is expected.

Tumor viability

Transarterial chemoembolization and focal tumor ablation (radiofrequency, ethanol, microwave, hot saline, and so forth) have been used for local tumor control of primary HCC and some metastatic liver tumors. Contrast-enhanced CT or contrast-enhanced MR imaging has traditionally been used to evaluate tumor viability and the role of ultrasound was limited before introduction of contrast agents [22,23]. Several reports describe the use of color or power Doppler to assess residual tumor flow [24,25]; however, these techniques lack sensitivity to slow flow and suffer from motion artifacts.

Unenhanced CT at 1 month following transarterial chemoembolization is useful for confirming successful accumulation of the radiopaque drug-carrying lipid emulsion into the targeted lesions. Although

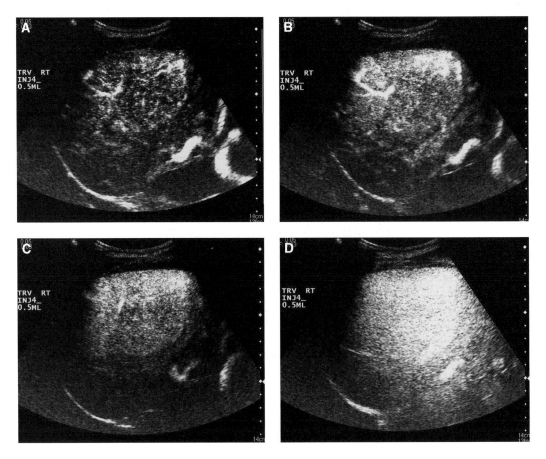

Fig. 5. Focal nodular hyperplasia with contrast-enhanced ultrasound. (*A* and *B*) A branching central artery with spoke-wheel appearance is seen (*arrow*) in the early arterial phase (angiographic phase) with low MI real-time imaging. (*C*) The lesion (*arrows*) enhances homogeneously and slightly more than liver indicative of a primary hepatic lesion with higher blood flow. (*D*) The lesion becomes isoechoic to hyperechoic compared with the surrounding liver on delayed imaging indicative of its benign characteristic.

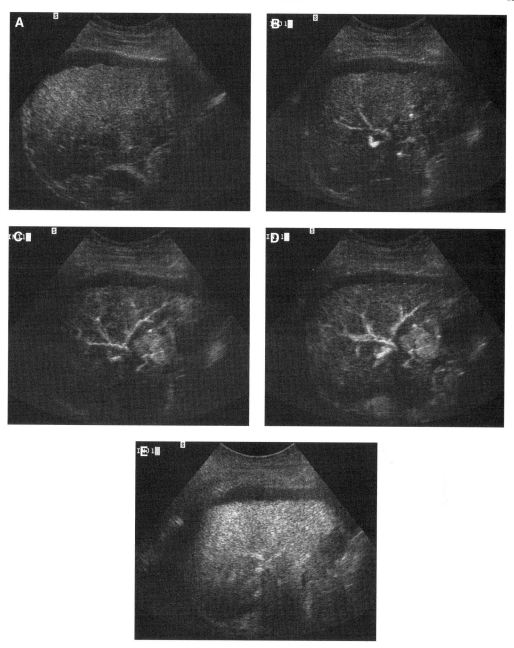

Fig. 6. Hepatocellular carcinoma with contrast-enhanced ultrasound. (*A*) Precontrast a hypoechoic tumor (*arrows*) is seen in the right lobe of the liver. (*B–E*) Contrast-enhanced ultrasound. Real-time images (*B* and *C*) show a feeding artery (*arrow*) and tumor blush in the early arterial phase. (*D*) Intermittent imaging with short delay shows homogenous enhancement of the whole tumor indicative of higher relative blood flow. (*E*) Long interval delay image shows the tumor (*arrows*) to be slightly hypoechoic compared with the surrounding liver suggesting its malignant nature.

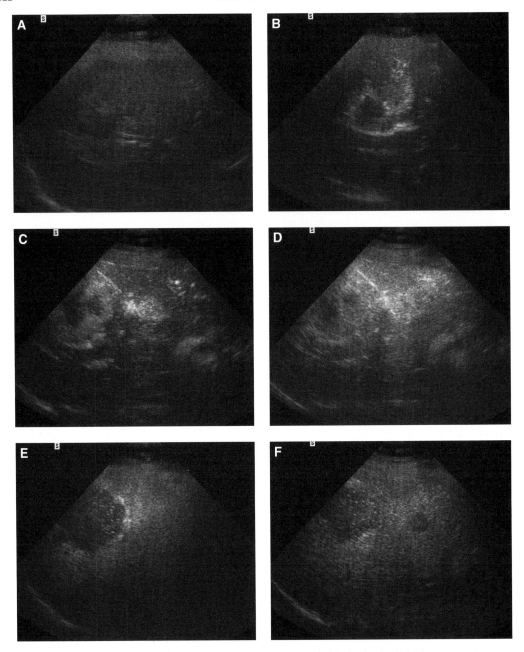

Fig. 7. Metastatic liver tumor from lung cancer with contrast-enhanced ultrasound. (*A*) Precontrast image. The tumor is subtle but slightly hypoechoic (*arrows*). (*B*) During real-time imaging, early filling of the tumor rim appeared (*arrows*) and became complete. (*C*) In addition, a smaller tumor became apparent (*arrows*) that was not seen before contrast. (*D*) With greater delay, the contrast agent filled the portal vein and enhanced the liver decreasing tumor contrast. (*E* and *F*) With greater delay-time, however, the liver became more echogenic than both metastatic lesions (*arrows*) because of the greater fractional blood volume and of the fact that microbubbles are slowed in the hepatic sinusoids.

Table 2
Differential diagnosis of hepatic tumors with contrast-enhanced ultrasound

Tumor	Arterial phase	Portal venous phase	Blood volume compared with normal liver	Late phase uptake[a]
HCC	Early diffuse enhancement	Early washout, iso- to hypoechoic	Iso- to low	No[b]
Metastasis	Early peripheral rim enhancement	Early washout, hypoechoic	Low	No
Hemangioma	Peripheral, nodular, and puddlelike appearance	Centripetal progression	High	Yes
FNH	Central artery. Spoke wheel vessel and homogeneous early enhancement from inside out	Hyperechoic with hypoechoic central scar	Iso- to high	Yes
Adenoma	Early entire enhancement from outside in	Hyperechoic and heterogeneous when large	Iso- to high	Yes

[a] With Levovist (see Ref. [16]).
[b] With exception of uptake in some well-differentiated HCC (see Ref. [38]).

contrast-enhanced CT is also used to detect residual blood flow, it is limited because the radiopaque lipid emulsion hides any subtle enhancement that may occur [23]. Lipiodol does not cause signal intensity changes on unenhanced MR imaging [26] allowing the detection of residual blood flow with contrast-enhanced MR imaging [23]. Unfortunately, because the small molecular weight water-soluble gadolinium agents diffuse throughout the extracellular fluid space, enhancement is also observed in posttreatment reactive granulation tissue decreasing specificity [27].

There are several studies evaluating the usefulness of contrast-enhanced ultrasound to assess the efficacy of focal tumor ablation [28–31], and their results are very promising. The advantages of contrast ultrasound are not only high spatial contrast and temporal resolution, but also the fundamental difference that microbubbles are pure intravascular agents. The high sensitivity of ultrasound to microbubbles allowing the visualization of a single microbubble [32] allows the recognition of perfused and viable tumor tissue.

Vascular imaging

Color and power Doppler technique has been improved and is sufficient to diagnose many vascular problems [33,34]. When the lesion is deep or there is not enough blood flow, however, it is still difficult to obtain confident diagnoses. Contrast agents enhance Doppler signals significantly and second harmonic technique has improved Doppler imaging by decreasing flash artifacts generated from non–contrast-containing pulsatile perivascular tissues and by limiting color to regions filled with bubbles [35]. These techniques do not overcome the limitations

of Doppler, however, such as unreliable filling of vessels, poor spatial resolution of color, and poor temporal resolution of power Doppler. Harmonic imaging with gray scale improves on standard gray-scale imaging by increasing contrast between the lumen and surrounding tissues. Gray scale filling of vessels is more powerful than filling the vessel with Doppler signal because the latter relies on flow to fill vessels and to provide anatomic detail.

In liver imaging, contrast-enhanced ultrasound is useful in evaluating the patency of transjugular intrahepatic portosystemic shunt [36], vascular complications post liver transplantation, and so forth.

Transit time analysis

Analysis of liver transit time of a bolus of ultrasound contrast agent, originally and mainly with Levovist, provides useful information about hemodynamic changes in patients with cirrhosis. Measurement of the arrival time of the bolus to the hepatic vein allows discrimination of patients with cirrhosis from controls and from patients with noncirrhotic diffuse liver disease, and has potential as a noninvasive test for cirrhosis [12,37]. The test in brief consists of injecting a bolus of Levovist intravenously and continuously monitoring the spectral Doppler signal in a hepatic vein from 20 seconds before the injection to 3 minutes afterward. The intensity of the spectral Doppler signal was measured to determine arrival time of the contrast agent by time–intensity curve analysis.

The normal volunteers and noncirrhotic patients showed very similar enhancement curves: the arrival times were late, and there was no significant differ-

Arrival Time

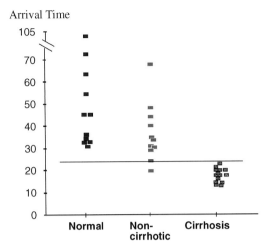

Fig. 8. Distribution of the arrival times in normal volunteers, patients with chronic liver disease, and cirrhotic patients. All patients with cirrhosis had an arrival time of less than 24 seconds, whereas all the normal volunteers and all but one of the noncirrhotic patients showed an arrival time of 24 seconds or more. (*Adapted from* Albrecht T, Blomley MJ, Cosgrove DO, et al. Non-invasive diagnosis of hepatic cirrhosis by transit-time analysis of an ultrasound contrast agent. Lancet 1999;353(9164):1579–83; with permission.)

ence. The cirrhotic patients showed a much earlier arrival time with an average of approximately 18 seconds, however, and this time was significantly different from the times of both the other two groups ($P < .001$ for both). Fig. 8 shows the distribution of the arrival times. It was determined that a 24-second arrival time from the time of injection or shorter discriminated cirrhotic patients from normal volunteers and all but one of the noncirrhotic patients [12]. It was also found that the more severe cirrhotic patients had even shorter arrival times (Fig. 9) [37]. This observation is based on the known arterialization of the liver and the development of intrahepatic shunt that occurs with cirrhosis.

Summary

Ultrasound contrast agents and contrast-specific imaging technology has greatly changed liver ultrasound. With contrast agents, ultrasound has become competitive with CT and MR imaging in lesion detection and may be even superior in lesion characterization and assessment of tumor viability following focal therapy. Moreover, ultrasound imaging main-

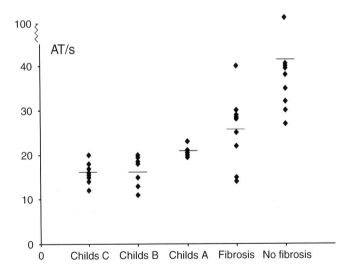

Fig. 9. Hepatic vein transit time plotted against diagnosis as a scatterplot, with mean values indicated as a horizontal line. The differences were highly significant ($P < .001$) using an ANOVA comparison. A hepatic vein transit time < 24 seconds and a carotid delay time (not shown) < 10 seconds were 100% sensitive for cirrhosis, but not completely specific. Two subjects with fibrosis had a carotid delay time < 10 seconds and three had a hepatic vein transit time < 24 seconds. (*Adapted from* Blomley MJ, Lim AK, Harvey CJ, et al. Liver microbubble transit time compared with histology and Child-Pugh score in diffuse liver disease: a cross sectional study. Gut 2003;53(8):118–93; with permission.)

tains its advantage of being portable, inexpensive, and real time.

Ultrasound contrast media are as critical in clinical practice as contrast media are for CT and MR imaging. The ability clearly to visualize vessels in solid tissue and distinguish vascular from nonvascular structures should make it easy to distinguish solid lesions from complex cysts, inflammation from abscess formation, hypervascular from hypovascular tumors, and so forth. With alteration in transmit power or intermittent imaging, image contrast can be manipulated to display vessels or tissue enhancement to highlight regions with different blood flow or fractional blood volume. These capabilities may prove superior to those of CT and MR imaging and will be available at the bedside or intraoperatively.

References

[1] Daniele B, Bencivenga A, Megna AS, et al. Alpha-fetoprotein and ultrasonography screening for hepatocellular carcinoma. Gastroenterology 2004;127: S108–12.

[2] Gramiak R, Shah PM. Echocardiography of the aortic root. Invest Radiol 1968;3:356–66.

[3] Mattrey RF, Scheible FW, Gosink BB, et al. Perfluoroctylbromide: a liver/spleen-specific and tumor-imaging ultrasound contrast material. Radiology 1982;145: 759–62.

[4] Parker KJ, Tuthill TA, Lerner RM, et al. A particulate contrast agent with potential for ultrasound imaging of liver. Ultrasound Med Biol 1987;13:555–66.

[5] Mattrey RF, Strich G, Shelton RE, et al. Perfluorochemicals as US contrast agents for tumor imaging and hepatosplenography: preliminary clinical results. Radiology 1987;163:339–43.

[6] Mattrey RF, Steinbach G, Lee Y, et al. High-resolution harmonic gray-scale imaging of normal and abnormal vessels and tissues in animals. Acad Radiol 1998; 5(Suppl 1):S63–5 [discussion: S64–72].

[7] Miller AP, Nanda NC. Contrast echocardiography: new agents. Ultrasound Med Biol 2004;30:425–34.

[8] Wilson SR, Burns PN. Liver mass evaluation with ultrasound: the impact of microbubble contrast agents and pulse inversion imaging. Semin Liver Dis 2001; 21:147–59.

[9] Quaia E, Stacul F, Bertolotto M, et al. Characterization of focal liver lesions with pulse inversion harmonic imaging (PIHI) using a second generation US contrast agent. Acad Radiol 2002;9(Suppl 2):S376–9.

[10] Strobel D, Raeker S, Martus P, et al. Phase inversion harmonic imaging versus contrast-enhanced power Doppler sonography for the characterization of focal liver lesions. Int J Colorectal Dis 2003;18:63–72.

[11] Kono Y, Steinbach GC, Peterson T, et al. Mechanism of parenchymal enhancement of the liver with a microbubble-based US contrast medium: an intravital microscopy study in rats. Radiology 2002;224:253–7.

[12] Albrecht T, Blomley MJ, Cosgrove DO, et al. Non-invasive diagnosis of hepatic cirrhosis by transit-time analysis of an ultrasound contrast agent. Lancet 1999; 353:1579–83.

[13] Burns PN. Instrumentation for contrast echocardiography. Echocardiography 2002;19:241–58.

[14] Sirlin CB, Girard MS, Baker KG, et al. Effect of acquisition rate on liver and portal vein enhancement with microbubble contrast. Ultrasound Med Biol 1999; 25:331–8.

[15] Wilson SR, Burns PN, Muradali D, et al. Harmonic hepatic US with microbubble contrast agent: initial experience showing improved characterization of hemangioma, hepatocellular carcinoma, and metastasis. Radiology 2000;215:153–61.

[16] Bryant TH, Blomley MJ, Albrecht T, et al. Improved characterization of liver lesions with liver-phase uptake of liver-specific microbubbles: prospective multicenter study. Radiology 2004;232:799–809.

[17] Quaia E, Calliada F, Bertolotto M, et al. Characterization of focal liver lesions with contrast-specific US modes and a sulfur hexafluoride-filled microbubble contrast agent: diagnostic performance and confidence. Radiology 2004;232:420–30.

[18] Freeny PC, Marks WM. Patterns of contrast enhancement of benign and malignant hepatic neoplasms during bolus dynamic and delayed CT. Radiology 1986;160:613–8.

[19] Honda H, Matsuura Y, Onitsuka H, et al. Differential diagnosis of hepatic tumors (hepatoma, hemangioma, and metastasis) with CT: value of two-phase incremental imaging. AJR Am J Roentgenol 1992;159: 735–40.

[20] Quillin SP, Atilla S, Brown JJ, et al. Characterization of focal hepatic masses by dynamic contrast-enhanced MR imaging: findings in 311 lesions. Magn Reson Imaging 1997;15:275–85.

[21] Sirlin CB, Lee YZ, Girard MS, et al. Contrast-enhanced B-mode US angiography in the assessment of experimental in vivo and in vitro atherosclerotic disease. Acad Radiol 2001;8:162–72.

[22] Kim SK, Lim HK, Kim YH, et al. Hepatocellular carcinoma treated with radio-frequency ablation: spectrum of imaging findings. Radiographics 2003;23:107–21.

[23] Kubota K, Hisa N, Nishikawa T, et al. Evaluation of hepatocellular carcinoma after treatment with trans-catheter arterial chemoembolization: comparison of Lipiodol-CT, power Doppler sonography, and dynamic MRI. Abdom Imaging 2001;26:184–90.

[24] Sumi S, Yamashita Y, Mitsuzaki K, et al. Power Doppler sonography assessment of tumor recurrence after chemoembolization therapy for hepatocellular carcinoma. AJR Am J Roentgenol 1999;172:67–71.

[25] Hosoki T, Yosioka Y, Matsubara T, et al. Power Doppler sonography of hepatocellular carcinoma treated by transcatheter arterial chemoembolization: assessment of the therapeutic effect. Acta Radiol 1999;40:639–43.

[26] De Santis M, Alborino S, Tartoni PL, et al. Effects of lipiodol retention on MRI signal intensity from hepatocellular carcinoma and surrounding liver treated by chemoembolization. Eur Radiol 1997;7:10–6.

[27] Kuszyk BS, Boitnott JK, Choti MA, et al. Local tumor recurrence following hepatic cryoablation: radiologic-histopathologic correlation in a rabbit model. Radiology 2000;217:477–86.

[28] Cioni D, Lencioni R, Bartolozzi C. Percutaneous ablation of liver malignancies: imaging evaluation of treatment response. Eur J Ultrasound 2001;13:73–93.

[29] Ding H, Kudo M, Onda H, et al. Evaluation of post-treatment response of hepatocellular carcinoma with contrast-enhanced coded phase-inversion harmonic US: comparison with dynamic CT. Radiology 2001; 221:721–30.

[30] Solbiati L, Ierace T, Tonolini M, et al. Guidance and monitoring of radiofrequency liver tumor ablation with contrast-enhanced ultrasound. Eur J Radiol 2004;51:S19–23.

[31] Kono Y, Alton K, Rose S, et al. Early assessment of treatment success with contrast-enhanced ultrasound post transarterial chemoembolization for hepatocellular carcinoma [abstract 385]. Radiological Society of North America 90th Scientific Assembly and Annual Meeting. Chicago, Illinois, November 27–December 2, 2004.

[32] Klibanov AL, Rasche PT, Hughes MS, et al. Detection of individual microbubbles of ultrasound contrast agents: imaging of free-floating and targeted bubbles. Invest Radiol 2004;39:187–95.

[33] Zwiebel WJ. Sonographic diagnosis of hepatic vascular disorders. Semin Ultrasound CT MR 1995;16: 34–48.

[34] Kruskal JB, Newman PA, Sammons LG, et al. Optimizing Doppler and color flow US: application to hepatic sonography. Radiographics 2004;24:657–75.

[35] Burns PN, Powers JE, Fritzsch T. Harmonic imaging: new imaging and Doppler method for contrast-enhanced ultrasound. Radiology 1992;185(P):142.

[36] Kono Y, Mattrey R, Pinnell S, et al. Ultrasound contrast venography of TIPS: gray-scale ultrasound vs. x-ray venography. J Ultrasound Med 2001;20(3):S82.

[37] Blomley MJK, Lim AKP, Harvey CJ, et al. Liver microbubble transit time compared with histology and Child-Pugh score in diffuse liver disease: a cross sectional study. Gut 2003;52:1188–93.

[38] Kitamura H, Kawasaki S, Nakajima K, et al. Correlation between microbubble contrast-enhanced color Doppler sonography and immunostaining for Kupffer cells in assessing the histopathologic grade of hepatocellular carcinoma: preliminary results. J Clin Ultrasound 2002;30:465–71.

ELSEVIER
SAUNDERS

Radiol Clin N Am 43 (2005) 827–848

RADIOLOGIC
CLINICS
of North America

Multidetector Row CT of the Liver

Aytekin Oto, MD[a],*, Eric P. Tamm, MD[b], Janio Szklaruk, MD, PhD[b]

[a]Department of Radiology, University of Texas Medical Branch at Galveston, 2.815 John Sealy Annex,
301 University Boulevard, Galveston, TX 77555, USA
[b]Department of Diagnostic Radiology, MD Anderson Cancer Center, University of Texas, 1515 Holcombe Boulevard, Box 57,
Houston, TX 77030, USA

CT has always played a major role in the imaging of the liver. Recent advances in MR imaging and ultrasound, such as three-dimensional high-resolution sequences, parallel imaging techniques, and new contrast agents, have helped to increase their popularity and use [1,2]. Nevertheless, the development of multidetector row CT (MDCT) technology has helped CT to continue to excel in its already established indications (ie, hepatic lesion detection and characterization) and to add new clinical indications (ie, CT angiography for preprocedure mapping, liver perfusion) [3–6]. The fast pace of development challenged radiologists in terms of the cost of replacement of scanners, the optimization of CT protocols for existing indications, and the development of new protocols for the new applications introduced by the MDCT technology.

This article discusses the advantages of MDCT for liver imaging, suggests guidelines to improve image quality through optimizing scanning protocols and contrast administration strategies, and reviews the potential clinical applications.

Multidetector row CT technology

Evolution of multidetector row CT technology

The concept of simultaneous multiple acquisitions per each gantry rotation was first introduced with dual-slice CT scanners in 1992 [7]. The first major development in MDCT technology, however, was the introduction of four-slice multidetector row scanners in 1998. Four-slice scanning protocols were primarily focused on optimization of existing single-slice helical CT parameters, such as slice thickness and table speed. With the development of systems with a higher number of detector rows (8, 10, and 16) in 2001 and 2002, there has been a shift toward isometric imaging (voxels of identical dimension in all three planes). The subsequent introduction of 32-, 40-, and 64-slice scanners at the 2003 Radiological Society of North America meeting showed the rapid pace of development of MDCT. In addition to the increase in the number of detector arrays from 4 to 64, rotation speed has decreased down to 0.33 seconds, tube efficiency has increased, and data handling capacity and image reconstruction techniques have improved.

Advantages of multidetector row CT

The main advantage MDCT has over single-slice spiral CT is speed. This can be used to decrease scan duration, increase distance of coverage, or increase resolution in the z-axis. In liver imaging, faster scanning decreases respiration artifacts and improves multiphase imaging. With the newest systems, it is possible to obtain images from multiple phases of hepatic contrast enhancement during the same breath-hold. This may facilitate digital subtraction of precontrast images from postcontrast images improving the various features of contrast enhancement. This has also made possible true quantitative perfusion studies of the liver [8–10].

* Corresponding author.
E-mail address: ayoto@utmb.edu (A. Oto).

Thinner slice collimation and isotropic volumetric imaging

MDCT scanners permit acquisition of thin slices with isotropic voxel size. A four-detector scanner can cover the entire liver in 10 seconds with a collimation of 1.25 mm. With a 16-detector scanner the collimation can be decreased to 0.625 mm, and with a 64-detector scanner it is possible to cover the liver with isotropic slices of 0.4 mm resolution in less than 5 seconds. The advantages of thinner, isotropic slices are less partial volume averaging and, more importantly, superior quality multiplanar reconstructions (MPR) and true isotropic three-dimensional reconstructions.

There have been controversial data in the literature about the role of thin-slice imaging for the detection and characterization of liver lesions. Initially, Weg and coworkers [11] reported improved liver lesion detection with greater conspicuity using a dual-detector scanner with 2.5-mm collimation compared with 5- and 7.5-mm collimation. Subsequently, however, Haider and coworkers [12] and then Kawata and coworkers [13] demonstrated that slice thickness less than 5 mm did not improve detection of liver metastases or hepatocellular carcinoma (HCC). Currently, no published large series addresses the effect of submillimeter collimation thickness on lesion detection using 16- and 64-detector scanners. Submillimeter isotropic images, however, have the potential to characterize small lesions in the liver better by providing accurate information about their enhancement pattern, feeding vessels, and perfusion.

Multiplanar and three-dimensional reconstructions

Thick MPRs (2–5 mm) of axial, coronal, or arbitrarily angulated sections derived from raw data obtained by very thin (submillimeter) effective collimation thickness could potentially be a primary mode for image review. Superior quality MPRs obtained in various planes may ultimately improve the detection of small subcapsular lesions, can show the feeding arteries and venous drainage of detected lesions, or help in the characterization of lesions by better demonstrating their enhancement patterns. Examples include peripheral nodules of enhancement of small hemangiomas or central scars in focal nodular hyperplasia [14–16]. The improved z-axis resolution of MDCT decreases stair-step artifact in reconstructed images. In addition, the anatomic coronal plane is preferred by surgeons for preoperative planning, because the relationship of the lesions to the blood vessels and bile ducts is better delineated [3]. Multiplanar volume rendering and creation of maximum intensity projections from MDCT data allow evaluation of both parenchymal and vascular detail in real time, interactively, with infinite viewing projections.

CT angiography images can be created through three-dimensional reconstructions of the thin-slice, isotropic images obtained in the early hepatic-arterial phase during a breathhold of 5 to 15 seconds. Maximum intensity projection, surface-shaded display, and volume-rendered techniques have been applied to the production of CT angiography to depict vascular anatomy (Fig. 1) [3]. CT angiography enables surgeons to understand the anatomy of the celiac trunk, hepatic arteries, and hepatic and portal venous system before liver resection or transplantation and helps in the planning of chemoembolization and surgical implantation of chemotherapy catheters by depicting the anatomy of the gastroduodenal artery and the origins of the proper hepatic and right and left hepatic arteries (Fig. 2) [3–6,17–21]. Additional significant information obtained from these images includes celiac axis stenosis, diameter of inflow arterial vessels, splenic artery aneurysms, and segmental involvement of tumor. CT angiography also plays a role in the setting of post–liver transplantation in the detection of hepatic arterial complications [22].

MDCT portal venography can display the entire portal venous system and help determine the extent and location of portosystemic collateral vessels in patients with portal hypertension [18,20]. Multiplanar images can detect and identify all major variations of the hepatic venous confluence and portal venous trifurcation (see Fig. 2).

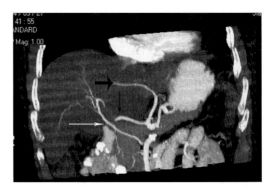

Fig. 1. A 72-year-old man with HCC. Maximum intensity projection reconstructed from the axial MDCT images obtained during the early arterial phase of contrast enhancement demonstrates anatomic variant of the hepatic artery. There is a left hepatic artery from the left gastric artery (*thick black arrow*). There is an accessory right hepatic artery from the superior mesenteric artery (*white arrow*). The hepatic artery from the celiac artery is also seen (*thin black arrow*).

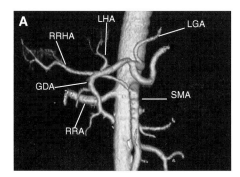
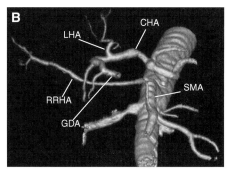
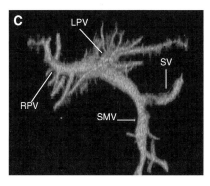

Fig. 2. Volume-rendered CT arteriogram, created with a seed-growing algorithm, shows in the coronal (*A*) and inferior oblique (*B*) projections variant origin of the right hepatic artery (RRHA) from the superior mesenteric artery (SMA). CT portogram (*C*) similarly created from same patient shows splenic vein (SV), superior mesenteric vein (SMV), and left (LPV) and right (RPV) portal veins and their segmental branches. CHA, common hepatic artery; LHA, left hepatic artery; GDA, gastroduodenal artery; RRA, right renal artery; and LGA, left gastric artery.

Minimum intensity image reconstructions allow for evaluation of biliary tree anatomy (Fig. 3). Minimum intensity reconstructions can detect biliary strictures, anatomic variants, or masses. The authors' protocol uses 2-mm coronal oblique minimum intensity reconstructions to improve evaluation of the extrahepatic biliary system and 10-mm coronal oblique minimum intensity reconstructions for evaluation of the intrahepatic bile ducts.

Virtual hepatectomy with volume-rendered images and liver volume estimation before surgery is useful in planning the extent and nature of hepatic resection [23]. Estimation of liver volume using three-dimensional techniques, when combined with clinical and laboratory evaluation of liver function, can facilitate the prediction of postoperative liver failure in patients undergoing resection, assist in embolization procedures, and aid planning of staged hepatic resection for bilobar disease (Fig. 4).

The review of CT angiography, minimum intensity, volume-rendered, and the axial source images can provide essential information for liver lesion characterization, staging, and biliary and vascular

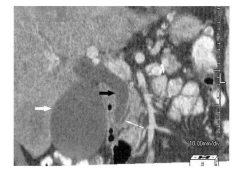

Fig. 3. A 71-year-old man with neuroendocrine tumor. Minimum intensity projection images of the hilar region reconstructed from the axial CT images obtained during the portal venous phase of contrast enhancement demonstrates a prominent bile duct (*black arrow*), gallbladder (*thick white arrow*), and pancreatic duct (*thin white arrow*). There is a stricture at the distal common bile duct.

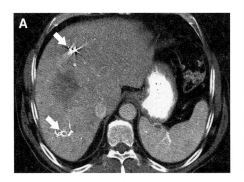
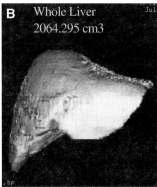
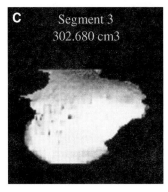

Fig. 4. A 58-year-old woman with a neuroendocrine tumor metastatic to the liver. (*A*) Axial MDCT image of the abdomen obtained during the late phase of contrast enhancement. The portal vein coils to the right. Portal vein branches are visualized (*arrows*). (*B*) Volume-rendered image of the whole liver with an estimated total liver volume of 2064 mL. (*C*) Volume-rendered image of segment III with an estimated volume of 303 mL.

mapping. A single-stop CT examination can provide all the information necessary for planning partial liver resection or liver transplantation.

Multiphase scanning

With single-slice helical CT, multiphase imaging of the liver included a hepatic-arterial phase and a portal-venous phase, which start 20 to 25 seconds and 60 to 70 seconds after the beginning of intravenous contrast material injection, respectively. After the advent of MDCT, different phases of hepatic enhancement were better defined, and accurate temporal localization of scanning has become more crucial (Fig. 5). Foley and coworkers [24] further divided the hepatic-arterial phase into early and late arterial phases. Early arterial phase, which is termed "the arterial phase" by Foley and coworkers [24], begins at the peak of aortic enhancement (approximately 15 seconds after initiating the bolus) and lasts for about 7 to 12 seconds. During this phase, there is mainly enhancement in the hepatic artery and its branches with little or no hepatic parenchymal en-

hancement (Fig. 6A). Late arterial phase starts approximately 30 seconds after initiation of the contrast bolus and again lasts for about 12 seconds. During this phase there is still arterial enhancement, early portal venous and hepatic parenchymal enhancement, but no hepatic venous enhancement (Fig. 6B). Foley and coworkers [24] concluded that although the early arterial phase was advantageous for CT angiography, it was not useful to detect hypervascular tumors [24]. In that study, maximum tumor-to-liver contrast was observed in the late arterial phase (portal inflow phase) in patients with and without cirrhosis. These findings were initially challenged by the results of a study by Murakami and coworkers [25], which showed that a combination of both early and late arterial-phase imaging resulted in improved detection. Several other studies comparing these two phases, however, later supported and confirmed the results of the study by Foley and coworkers [26–29]. Even though the early arterial phase did not show any improvement in the detection of hypervascular masses, it may still have the potential for improving

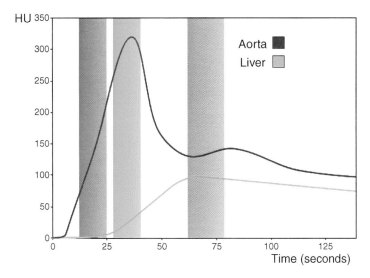

Fig. 5. Graph shows different phases of hepatic enhancement (early arterial [purple], late arterial [green], and portal venous phases [orange]) that can be obtained by MDCT.

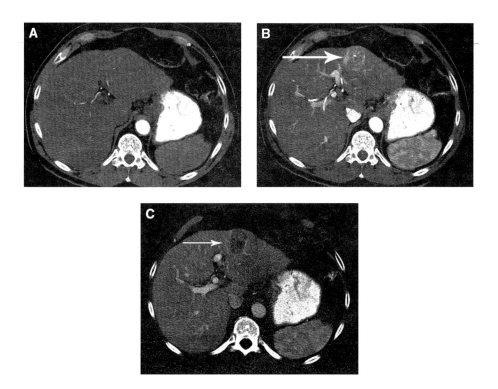

Fig. 6. MDCT evaluation of the abdomen of a 65-year-old man obtained during the early arterial (*A*), late arterial (*B*), and late portal venous phases of enhancement (*C*). There is a hypervascular mass in the left lobe of the liver that has increased enhancement during the late arterial phase of contrast administration *(B, arrow)*. The mass is hypoattenuating and demonstrates a hyperattenuating capsule on delayed images (*C, arrow*).

832   OTO et al

characterization of these lesions through identifying feeding vessels and improving depiction of tumor vascular architecture.

The third phase, which is traditionally known as the "portal-venous phase" (also termed "hepatic-venous phase" by Foley and coworkers [24]) begins about 45 seconds after the beginning of the early arterial phase (approximately 60–70 seconds after the initiation of bolus) and represents the peak of hepatic parenchymal and portal-venous enhancement together with opacification of hepatic veins (Fig. 6C). As in single-slice scanning, the portal-venous phase (60–70 seconds) is the ideal phase for detection of hypovascular liver lesions in MDCT protocols [24,29]. A fourth delayed phase, which is also termed the "equilibrium phase," can be obtained 90 to 120 seconds after the start of administration of intravenous contrast and may be helpful in better delineation of certain pathologies, such as cholangiocarcinoma and some HCCs [30,31].

Limitations of multidetector row CT

Handling and interpretation of the large number of data sets acquired by MDCT scanners still remains a major challenge despite advances in reconstruction speed, improved rates of image transfer, and availability of inexpensive and large-scale data storage. Another limitation of MDCT is worsening image noise with reduced slice thickness. Reconstructing thicker MPR and three-dimensional reconstruction images can help to reduce image noise. Finally,

increased scanning speed results in more sharply defined hepatic phases; this requires more precise timing of scanning.

Future applications

Tumor angiogenesis has significant implications in the diagnosis and treatment of a variety of malignancies. With current MDCT scanners, both tissue and vascular enhancement can be measured and traced at small intervals, allowing calculation of quantitative angiogenesis parameters, such as tissue blood flow, blood volume, mean transit time, contrast arrival time, and the arterial fraction of hepatic perfusion [32]. Perfusion data can help assessment of the degree of chronic liver disease, early detection of metastases, characterization of liver lesions, and response of metastatic lesions to treatment (Fig. 7) [9,10,32]. Further research with MDCT can better demonstrate the impact of this new technology.

Guidelines for multidetector row CT liver protocols

In MDCT protocols, slice collimation, effective slice thickness, table speed, and reconstruction increment are the most important acquisition and reconstruction parameters (Table 1). Effective slice thickness can be determined after the acquisition of data and the raw data can be reconstructed with an effective slice thickness different from collimation. For example, once data are acquired using 0.625-mm collimation by a 16-detector scanner (16 × 0.625 mm), the data can be reconstructed to any effective slice

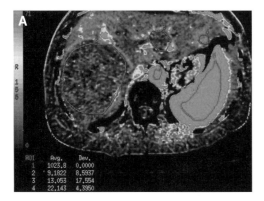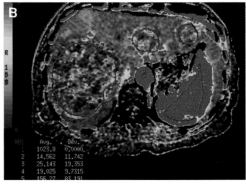

Fig. 7. Functional CT (blood flow) map of the liver obtained with CT two-perfusion software (GEMS, Milwaukee, Wisconsin) in a 65-year-old woman with metastatic carcinoid to the liver. CT blood flow map refers to functional CT data acquisition by a cine-CT mode and the application of the software developed by Ting-Yim Lee. (*A*) Blood flow (mL/min/100 g tissue) map at baseline. (*B*) Blood flow map at 48 hours following treatment with bevacizumab, a recombinant humanized monoclonal IgG antibody that neutralizes vascular endothelial growth factor and blocks the growth of new vessels. There is a decrease in blood flow. (*From* Miles KA, Charnsangavej C, Lee FT, et al. Application of CT in the investigation of angiogenesis in oncology. Acad Radiol 2000;7:840–50; with permission.)

Table 1
Sample protocols for 4- and 16-detector row CT scanners

Criteria	4-detector	16-detector
Detector collimation (mm)	1.25[a] and 2.5	0.63 and 1.25
Table speed and rotation (mm)	7.5[a] and 15	10[a] and 20
Pitch	1.5	~1
Effective slice thickness (mm)	1.25[a]–5	0.63[a] and 5
Reconstruction increment (mm)	1 and 5	0.63[a] and 5
kV(p)	120–140	120–140
Contrast concentration (mgI/mL)	370	370
Contrast volume (mL)	120–150	120–150
Timing	Bolus tracking for the early and late arterial phase Either bolus tracking or fixed delay of 65 seconds for portal venous phase	

[a] For three-dimensional and multiplanar reconstructions.

thickness equal to or greater than 0.625 mm. Slightly wider (25%–30%) effective slice thickness compared with slice collimation provides optimum signal-to-noise ratio. For MPR and three-dimensional reconstruction, the reconstruction increment should allow at least 60% overlap relative to the effective section thickness [33]. Urban and coworkers [34] have shown that overlapping reconstructions allow detection of more lesions in the liver than contiguous reconstructions. In MDCT, pitch is generally defined as the table travel per rotation divided by the collimation of the x-ray beam (number of channels times slice collimation) and has a smaller effect on image quality than it has with single-slice CT scanners [35,36].

Thin slices and fastest gantry rotation times are preferred in CT imaging of the liver [37]. Two different strategies of data acquisition and reconstruction have been used in MDCT liver protocols. The first strategy is to acquire the data with the thinnest possible collimation (1.25 mm in 4-detector scanners and 0.625 mm in 16-detector scanners) and then to reconstruct overlapping slices with either the same or slightly wider effective slice thickness. This secondary raw data set is used as source images of two-dimensional MPR and three-dimensional CT angiography reconstructions. The second data acquisition strategy is used to produce axial images for evaluation of the parenchyma. The data are acquired by relatively thick collimation (2.5 mm in 4-detector

scanners and 1.25–2 mm in 16-detector scanners) and then thicker, contiguous slices (2–5 mm) are reconstructed. With the advent of 16- and especially 64-detector scanners, the first strategy, which allows true isotropic volumetric imaging, is replacing the acquisition of thicker-collimation data sets and liver parenchyma can be evaluated by reviewing the relatively thick slice MPRs (2–5 mm) in various planes obtained from the thin-collimation (submillimeter) data sets.

Contrast material

The dual blood supply of the liver (25% from the hepatic artery and 75% from the portal vein) and the necessity for both good spatial and contrast resolution make the optimization of liver CT protocols challenging. As the scanning times get shorter, the duration of injections can potentially be decreased, and contrast material administration techniques need to be revised.

Concentration of iodine. Despite the ability to reduce the necessary contrast dose for MDCT angiography of the body, a decrease in the iodine dose has not been possible for MDCT imaging of the liver [38]. The reason is the direct relation of the enhancement magnitude of the liver to the amount of iodine delivered. There are two ways of delivering the same amount of iodine in a shorter time. The first is to administer a contrast material with a higher concentration of iodine and the other is to increase the injection rate. When Awai and coworkers [39] compared the effect of using different iodine concentrations (300 versus 370 mg/mL) of contrast material in liver CT, they concluded that higher concentration of iodine improved depiction of hypervascular HCCs and aortic enhancement during the arterial phase. There was no significant difference between the two groups in terms of hepatic enhancement at the arterial phase and tumor-to-liver contrast in the portal-venous phase. In another study, Furuta and coworkers [40] showed that higher iodine concentration (370 mg/mL) contrast medium can lead to better enhancement of the liver in the portal-venous phase and also improves overall image quality and diagnostic accuracy. Similar or better results with smaller volumes while using higher-concentration contrast material can also lead to potential cost savings because the price of the contrast generally varies by volume.

Contrast injection. The second way to administer the same amount of iodine in a shorter time is to increase the injection rate. Increased injection rate also leads to better separation of arterial and portal-venous phases. There are physiologic limits, however, to how rapidly contrast media can be safely administered (5–6 mL/s maximum). As the rate of injection increases, the degree of contrast enhancement increases and the duration of contrast enhancement decreases [41,42]. This is especially important for aortic and hepatic arterial enhancement, whereas hepatic enhancement is relatively unaffected by an increase in flow rate [42].

The use of a saline flush following contrast injection was originally described by Hopper and coworkers [43] for thoracic spiral CT in 1997 but became popularized with the recent advent of double-barrel injectors. These injectors are equipped with two syringes, one for saline and one for contrast. By pushing the remaining contrast material in the injection tubing and possibly aiding propulsion of contrast in the venous system, saline flushing reduces contrast waste, allowing for a decrease in the net volume of contrast medium used without resulting in a significant decrease in the hepatic enhancement or lesion conspicuity [44]. This leads to cost savings and improved patient safety by decreasing the risk of nephrotoxicity [45].

Patient-related factors alter contrast-enhancement dynamics, and their influence can be more profound with short injections. Patient weight is the most important of these factors and is inversely related to the magnitude of hepatic enhancement [46]. Lower cardiac output delays both aortic and hepatic enhancement and leads to increased peak aortic enhancement but does not have significant effect on the magnitude of hepatic enhancement [47].

Scan timing

There are three strategies to determine the timing of the scanning: (1) fixed delay time, (2) test bolus injection, and (3) bolus triggering. For CT angiography of the liver either test bolus injection or bolus triggering is necessary to customize the delay time for each patient. The early arterial-phase scan for CT angiography is started at the time of peak aortic enhancement or at aortic enhancement of arbitrary numbers between 100 and 150 HU [24,35]. If only two passes are planned through the liver (late arterial and portal venous), then the late arterial-phase scan can be triggered following a delay of 10 seconds after peak aortic enhancement time [27,48]. For a single portal-venous phase scan, a region of interest can be placed over the liver parenchyma and the scan can be triggered at 30 to 55 HU hepatic enhancement over the baseline. Using fixed delay times (ie, 30 seconds for late arterial phase and 60–70 seconds for portal-venous phase) does not take into account patient-related factors, such as weight and cardiac output. In

patients without circulatory disturbances, however, they can still be used. Itoh and coworkers [49] reported that the use of automatic bolus tracking in late arterial- and portal-venous phase hepatic CT did not significantly improve the degree of contrast enhancement of the liver or lesion conspicuity in patients without circulatory disturbances.

Radiation issues

Clinical scan parameters should be optimized to achieve a balance between radiation dose and image quality. Scanning with thinner-slice collimation, over-beaming (wider beam collimation compared with detector size along the z-axis), and multiphase scanning with increased number of phases can cause an increase in the radiation dose. Recently developed prepatient filtration and collimation of the x-ray beam, automatic modulation of tube current in all three dimensions, and various dose-reduction filters help to reduce radiation exposure [50,51]. Changing the tube potential (kilovolt [peak] [kV[p]) and current (milliamperes) according to the patient's weight and cross-sectional dimensions can lead to reduced radiation exposure to lighter patients without impairing image quality [51].

The radiation dose increases exponentially with increasing kilovolt (peak). The effect of tube voltage on image quality is complex. Reduction in tube potential leads to increased noise but improves tissue contrast [50]. In liver protocols, a tube potential of 120 kV(p) is usually preferred. An increase to 140 kV(p) may be considered in large patients.

The relationship between tube current and radiation dose is linear. A reduction in tube current causes increase in image noise, which degrades low-contrast resolution. In some modern multislice CT scanners, the effective milliampere (milliampere per pitch) concept has been introduced where image noise can be kept constant by adjusting the milliampere while changing the pitch factor. Most current scanners combine both z-axis and angular tube current modulation to adjust the dose to the size and shape of the patient. In some scanners it is possible to select the desired image quality (noise index) and based on the scout, the scanner adjusts the milliampere to achieve the selected noise level.

Benign lesions of the liver

Neoplasms

Most benign hepatic neoplasms are discovered incidentally. Uncommonly, large benign hepatic lesions can be symptomatic because of mass effect or complications, such as hemorrhage. The most commonly encountered primary benign hepatic lesions are hepatic cysts, hemangioma, focal nodular hyperplasia, and hepatic adenoma. Uncommon benign primary hepatic neoplasms include biliary cystadenoma and fatty lesions, such as lipoma, myelolipoma, and angiomyolipoma.

Cysts

A recent study of 617 patients evaluated by spiral CT found an 18% incidence of simple hepatic cysts, with greater prevalence in older patients [52]. The incidence is markedly increased in the setting of autosomal-dominant polycystic kidney disease.

Cysts are typically asymptomatic. When sufficiently large, however, they can become symptomatic secondary to mass effect on adjacent structures. Extrinsic compression of the biliary tree has been reported [53].

Cysts typically measure water density (<20 HU); do not enhance; and have well-defined borders without perceptible walls (Fig. 8). Partial volume averaging of cysts with liver parenchyma, however, can result in mild increase in attenuation following the administration of intravenous contrast. Complications include hemorrhage and infection; these can also result in density measurements higher than that for simple fluid. MDCT allows for thin-section images to be obtained during peak hepatic enhancement in the portal-venous phase minimizing partial volume averaging artifact, while maximizing the detection of subtle enhancement in the case of cystic metastases or abscess.

The differential diagnosis of a hepatic cyst includes cystic metastases from cystic primary tumors (ovarian, cystic pancreatic primaries) and solid tumors that can produce cystic metastases (gastrointestinal

stromal tumor, endometrial carcinoma) [54,55]. Abscesses, secondary to bacterial or amebic infection, usually show peripheral wall enhancement but can mimic cysts especially when they are small [56,57]. Biliary cystadenoma-cystadenocarcinoma typically is a large lesion with nodularity, internal septations, and a perceptible wall [58].

Hemangioma

Hemangioma is the most common benign liver tumor with a frequency of up to 20% at autopsy [59]. They are typically asymptomatic, are usually found incidentally on CT, and can present as multiple lesions of variable size. Hemangiomas typically show early peripheral nodular enhancement with gradual filling over time, from the periphery to the central portion of the tumor (Fig. 9). The identification of globular enhancement that is isodense to the aorta allows discrimination of hemangiomas from metastases [60]. Small lesions often enhance uniformly even on early phases of imaging, however, and large lesions, such as giant hemangiomas (6–10 cm in size) may show persistent regions that do not enhance. Occasionally, hemangiomas may be associated with arterioportal shunting, which can result in confusion with metastatic lesion, especially in the case of small hemangiomas [61,62]. Imaging during multiple phases is important to identify the characteristic pattern of enhancement when possible. In cases where imaging findings are equivocal, further assessment with MR imaging, or a technetium-labeled red blood cell scan, may be necessary.

Focal nodular hyperplasia

Focal nodular hyperplasia is the second most common benign lesion of the liver with an incidence of approximately 8% [63]. It is seen most commonly in women and typically occurs as a solitary lesion

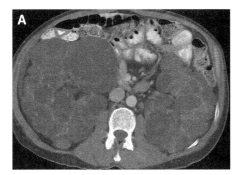
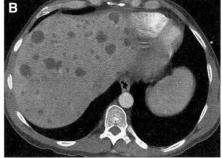

Fig. 8. A 48-year-old man with history of polycystic kidney disease. (*A*) Multiple cysts replace the renal parenchyma bilaterally. (*B*) Multiple hepatic cysts are also present.

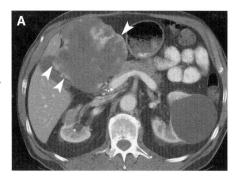
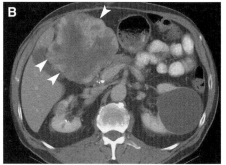

Fig. 9. A 74-year-old man with history of cavernous hemangioma. Globular regions of peripheral enhancement are identified (*arrowheads*) during the early arterial phase (*A*) and portal venous phase (*B*) with progressive enhancement peripherally.

(76%) with a size ranging from 1 mm to 19 cm in diameter [64].

The enhancement pattern on multiphase helical CT can be suggestive of the diagnosis. Focal nodular hyperplasia can be hypodense or isodense to the liver on precontrast images. It is typically hyperdense on arterial phase images (20–30 seconds after contrast injection) becoming less prominent on portal-venous phase images (70–90 seconds) and may become completely isodense to normal liver parenchyma (Fig. 10) [63]. About one third of cases show a central scar on imaging [65]. It typically is hypodense on precontrast and the arterial phase of imaging, becoming hyperdense on the portal-venous phase [63]. Unfortunately, focal nodular hyperplasia can show imaging characteristics suggestive of a primary or metastatic malignancy including rapid washout, persistent enhancement, absence of a central scar, or the presence of a capsule [66]. The primary differential is HCC, particularly fibrolamellar hepatoma, which can even mimic the appearance of the central scar. Hepatocyte-specific MR imaging agents or technetium sulfur colloid scans can be used in

problematic cases to differentiate metastatic disease from possible focal nodular hyperplasia, but are limited in their use because HCCs can also show Kupffer cell activity [67].

Hepatic adenoma

Hepatic adenoma is an uncommon benign tumor that is most commonly associated with oral contraceptives [68] and anabolic steroids [69] but has also been associated with glycogen storage disease [67]. Hepatic adenoma typically manifests as a solitary, encapsulated, well-defined, often hypervascular mass [67]. Hypervascularity is often best appreciated on a multiphase CT scan (Fig. 11) [70]. Findings on multiphasic CT, such as near uniform enhancement on portal-venous phase images, can help in suggesting a diagnosis [71]. Precontrast images may show low-density regions consistent with intratumoral fat, and high-density areas consistent with intratumoral hemorrhage [67]. The findings are often nonspecific and must be interpreted in the clinical context; tissue diagnosis may be necessary [72]. Large lesions are typically resected because of the possibility of hemor-

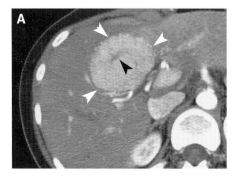
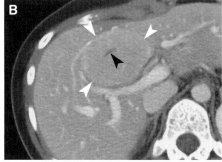

Fig. 10. A 22-year-old woman with history of focal nodular hyperplasia (*white arrowheads*) and central scar (*black arrowhead*) appearing hypervascular in the arterial phase (*A*) and isodense to the liver in the portal venous phase (*B*).

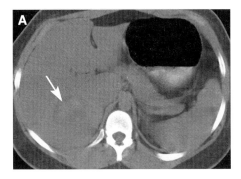
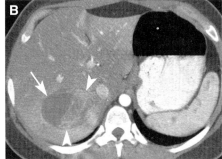
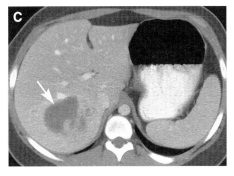

Fig. 11. A 25-year-old woman with biopsy-proved hepatic adenoma. Precontrast image (*A*) shows hyperdense region of hemorrhage (*arrow*). Early arterial phase image (*B*) shows regions of rapid enhancement (*arrowheads*). The region of hemorrhage (*arrow*) shows lack of enhancement on both the early arterial and portal venous (*C*).

rhage or rupture [73] and the small possibility of development of HCC [74]. The differential diagnosis for this lesion includes HCC, hypervascular metastases, and focal nodular hyperplasia.

Biliary cystadenoma

Biliary cystadenoma is a rare cystic neoplasm that arises from biliary epithelium. It is part of a continuum with biliary cystadenocarcinoma and is typically surgically resected because of the risk of malignant degeneration and because of the inability to differentiate benign from malignant lesions based on imaging [67,75,76]. Careful surgical technique is important because of the possibility of local recurrence [67]. Biliary cystadenocarcinoma can be divided into two groups based on the presence or absence of ovarian stroma; those with ovarian stroma are seen only in women and have a good prognosis [77].

These lesions are typically cystic, large lesions with septations (Fig. 12) and nodularity; the more prominent the septations and nodularity, the greater the likelihood of malignancy [78]. The regions of nodularity demonstrate enhancement, and calcifications may be present in the walls or septa [79].

The differential for this lesion includes other large cystic lesions, such as cystic metastases, large simple or complicated hepatic cysts, complex abscesses, echinococcal cysts, and intrahepatic biloma or hematoma [58,80,81]. Differentiation from complex-appearing lesions, such as complex abscesses and echinococcal cysts, may be difficult.

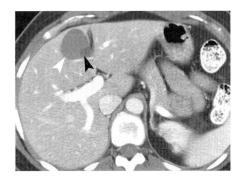

Fig. 12. A 44-year-old woman with history of biliary cystadenoma. Regions of relative hyperdensity (*white arrowhead*) and hypodensity (*black arrowhead*) are present within the lesion.

Focal inflammatory disease

Liver abscesses can result from a variety of infectious organisms. Integration of clinical signs and symptoms, laboratory values, and imaging findings can help in establishing a diagnosis, but often percutaneous aspiration is necessary to identify the causative organism.

Bacterial abscesses can result from hematogenous seeding, or from extension from the biliary tract. Imaging plays an important role in establishing diagnosis of abscess and guiding planning of percutaneous drainage. This is especially important because those who are at highest risk for mortality include the elderly with underlying malignancy that develop abscesses secondary to septicemia [82]; such patients can present with a complex clinical picture. Patients can have a single abscess, or multiple (Fig. 13). These lesions can be small (microabscesses) or large, even coalescing [83,84]. The use of intravenous contrast is vital to identifying abscesses [56]. The typical appearance is of a centrally hypodense lesion; a peripheral enhancing rim may be present but is not a sensitive sign [56,85]. Thin-section imaging during the portal-venous phase, as can be obtained with MDCT, can optimize detection of small abscesses and air bubbles that may be present within them [86].

In contrast, fungal abscesses typically occur in immunocompromised hosts. These typically manifest as microabscesses that involve the liver, spleen, and occasionally kidneys. They can occur secondary to a variety of organisms including cryptococcus, histoplasmosis, and mucormycosis, but most are secondary to *Candida albicans* [57,87]. Fungal abscesses

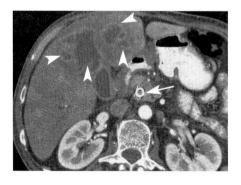

Fig. 13. A 70-year-old man with history of pancreatic cancer, status postchemotherapy with complication of sepsis and liver abscesses (*arrowheads*) with finger-like extensions into the liver parenchyma. Heterogeneous enhancement of the liver parenchyma during this early arterial-phase imaging is secondary to inflammation. Metallic wall stent (*arrow*) is also present.

typically have the appearance of multiple, small (2–20 mm), round, hypodense lesions that may or may not show peripheral enhancement [57]. CT is useful not only for the initial diagnosis, but also to evaluate for resolution with therapy.

Liver abscess is the most common extraintestinal complication of amebiasis, typically caused by the protozoan *Entamoeba histolytica*. Patients at presentation frequently have high fever and right upper quadrant pain. These abscesses are typically rounded, well-defined, lesions with relative low density, a perceptible enhancing wall typically associated with a peripheral hypodense zone representing edema. Septations, fluid-debris levels, and extrahepatic extension may be present [88].

Liver transplantation

MDCT plays a significant role in the work-up of transplant patients, both preoperatively and postoperatively. Preoperative imaging is best performed using a thin-section, multiphase (arterial and portal venous) technique with postprocessing to yield MDCT arteriograms. Dual-phase imaging optimizes the detection, localization, and determination of the extent of the most commonly encountered tumors (cholangiocarcinoma and HCC, particularly the latter) [89]. The sensitivity for HCC in cirrhotic patients awaiting transplant has been reported recently to be 79% [90]. Unfortunately, detection of lesions <2 cm is limited [90,91]. Preoperative imaging can determine the extrahepatic spread of disease, and identify complicating factors, such as portal vein thrombosis, varices, and ascites. MDCT can also be used to monitor for development of HCC in the cirrhotic patient awaiting transplant. Recent information suggests that as many as 20% of such patients who are negative at the time of initial listing as a transplant candidate can develop HCC while awaiting transplant [92].

Preoperative thin-section imaging and MDCT arteriograms can also detect important vascular abnormalities, including celiac stenosis, and aneurysms and pseudoaneurysms. Failure to recognize celiac stenosis and to ensure an adequate arterial blood supply to the liver can result acutely in hepatic necrosis, which can be fatal. Chronic ischemia from inadequate management of celiac stenosis can result in biliary strictures, cholangitis, and failure of the liver transplant [93]. Aneurysms, particularly of the splenic artery, are associated with significant postoperative complications [94]. MDCT arteriography is also useful to detect such anomalies as complete replacement of the common hepatic artery, with origin from the superior mesenteric artery; its usual

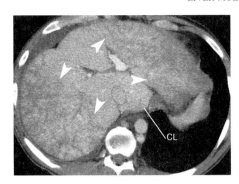

Fig. 14. A 33-year-old man with a history of colon cancer and Budd-Chiari syndrome. Peripheral hepatic congestion (*arrowheads*) and enlargement of the caudate (CL).

aberrant course posterior to the portal vein typically requires modification of the transplant procedure for creating a vascular anastomosis (see Fig. 2) [95]. MDCT has also been shown to be useful in assessment of relevant vascular anatomy for living related donor liver transplantation [5].

Postprocessing of thin-section CT data can also be used for evaluating other factors in the transplant recipient or donor. Recent data suggest that CT cholangiography can evaluate living potential liver donors for variant biliary anatomy, with results comparable with those of conventional MR cholanio-pancreatography (MRCP) and MRCP obtained with mangafodipir trisodium [96]. Postprocessing of MDCT data from the portal venous phase can be useful to detect hepatic venous variants that can impact right hepatectomy in living donor transplants [97]. Postprocessing is also useful for determining liver volumes for living (related) donors [98].

Ultrasound is typically used to evaluate for most complications in the postoperative period, including hepatic artery, portal vein, or inferior vena cava thrombosis or stenosis. CT is useful for the evaluation of such complications as abscess (intrahepatic or extrahepatic); extent of postoperative collections and their follow-up; extent of hepatic necrosis or intra-hepatic abscesses following hepatic artery thrombosis; hepatic artery pseudoaneurysms; and fluid collections secondary to bile leak [99]. CT can also incidentally identify thrombosis of the portal vein or inferior vena cava during the work-up of other complications [95]. Preliminary work with MDCT suggests that it may have a role in the assessment of posttransplant vascular complications, such as hepatic artery or portal vein stenosis [100,101].

MDCT is also useful for the detection of the late complication of tumors secondary to immunosuppressive therapy, typically non-Hodgkin's lymphomas or squamous cell skin cancers [95]. When lymphoma involves the transplanted liver, it can have the appearance of low-attenuation masses on CT, or porta hepatis masses encasing vasculature and the extrahepatic biliary ducts [102]. Recurrence of the patient's primary tumor can also sometimes occur [103].

Vascular disease

Budd-Chiari syndrome, obstruction of the liver's venous outflow, can occur in either acute or chronic forms. The former typically occurs in hypercoagulable states, as may occur in pregnancy, or tumor, with resulting obstruction of the inferior vena cava or main hepatic veins. The chronic form typically is secondary to fibrosis involving intrahepatic veins [104]. The typical appearance on CT examination is of a mottled enhancement pattern with delayed enhancement of the periphery of the liver, and compensatory enlargement of the caudate lobe (Fig. 14). The caudate lobe shows prominent enhancement compared with the remainder of the liver. Thrombosis of the intrahepatic veins or inferior vena cava may also be seen [105,106]. The differential diagnosis includes right-sided cardiac failure or congestive heart failure; however, enlargement of the hepatic veins differentiates these entities from Budd-Chiari syndrome [104].

Portal vein thrombosis can be acute or chronic, and can occur secondary to tumor invasion, external compression, or thrombosis from a variety of etiologies. Spiral CT has been used to improve detection of portal vein thrombosis [107]; it is expected that the thinner sections available with MDCT obtained at peak portal venous enhancement improve detection of acute thrombosis. The finding in acute thrombosis is a filling defect within the portal venous system

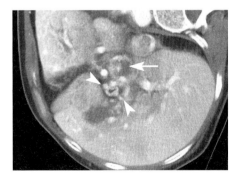

Fig. 15. A 53-year-old woman with history of HCC, showing portal vein thrombosis (*arrow*) and gallbladder varices (*arrowheads*).

(Fig. 15). Chronic findings include multiple periportal collateral vessels with ultimately development of cavernous transformation in which the portal vein is replaced by extensive collateral vessels [86].

MDCT also can detect perfusion defects, which can occur secondary to a variety of etiologies including secondary to tumor, thrombosis of segmental vascular branches, and vascular malformations. Careful analysis of the changes in the underlying liver parenchyma are necessary to exclude underlying tumor and close follow-up may be necessary. Thin-section imaging and postprocessing with MPR from MDCT may also play a role in demonstrating the complex anatomy of hepatic vascular malformations [108].

Malignant hepatic lesions

Primary hepatic malignancies

Hepatocellular carcinoma

HCC represents 6% of all cancers and is the most common primary hepatic malignancy worldwide. The most important risk factors include cirrhosis and hepatitis B and C viruses. There is a peak age incidence at 50 to 70 years with a 4:1 male predominance. HCC may present as a solitary mass, multifocal nodules, or diffuse disease throughout the liver. Pathologic features that may affect the imaging findings include the presence of a capsule, necrosis, calcifications, hemorrhage, fibrosis, or fat. The staging of HCC is based on TNM classification. The tumor (T) classification is based on the numbers of nodules present, the size of the nodules, and the presence of vascular invasion [109].

The most common clinical manifestations are ill-defined abdominal pain, weight loss, and hepatomegaly. Treatment options include surgery (resection or transplant); percutaneous regional therapy (percutaneous ethanol ablation, transarterial chemoembolization, cryoablation, or acetic acid injection); and systemic therapy (chemotherapy, immunotherapy, hormonal therapy, and radiation) [110]. Of the available therapies, surgery offers the best treatment option. Imaging plays an essential role in the clinical management of HCC with MDCT and MR imaging as the most commonly used imaging modality in the diagnosis, staging, and surveillance of the disease.

The postcontrast evaluation of the liver in patients suspected of HCC has evolved along with improvement in CT technology. The development of helical (spiral) CT technology made possible the implementation of a biphasic examination. This allowed for the acquisition of images during the late arterial phase and during the portal-venous phase of contrast enhancement [111].

This change in examination resulted in the finding of previously undetected hypervascular tumors that could only be visualized during the arterial-dominant phase of enhancement [111]. This is secondary to the abundant arterial neovascularity of HCC versus the portal venous-dominant vascular supply of normal liver parenchyma.

The typical CT appearance of HCC during a biphasic scan is an early enhancing mass with rapid washout on the late phase (see Fig. 6). A capsule, if present, demonstrates late enhancement (see Fig. 6). The biphasic technique has been shown to be more sensitive than single late-phase examination for the detection of HCC [111,112]. In one series, the combined review of the hepatic-arterial phase and the portal-venous phase detected 95% of lesions, whereas review of the portal-venous phase alone detected only 82% of lesions [111]. Oliver and coworkers [112] report that the combined review of hepatic-arterial phases and portal-venous phases detected 98% of lesions, whereas review of each phase alone detected 76% and 81% of lesions, respectively. These results show the combined review of both phases increases sensitivity for lesion detection.

The rapid evolution of MDCT has required revisions of imaging protocols to optimize detection of HCC. The authors' current MDCT protocol for evaluation of a patient with a clinical suspicion of HCC is an examination performed at these three stages of enhancement (see Fig. 6): (1) the early arterial phase at 15 seconds after the infusion of contrast, (2) the hepatic-arterial phase at 40 seconds, and (3) the portal-venous phase at 65 seconds after the infusion of contrast at 4 to 6 mL/s. The scan time for the entire liver is 10 to 12 seconds with a slice thickness of 2.5 to 5 mm and a pitch of 1.5. The images are reconstructed at 2.5-mm slice thickness. The hepatic-arterial phase has higher sensitivity than the early arterial phase and increases the sensitivity for detection of lesions less than 2 cm from 34% to 52%, to 79% to 82% [28]. For lesions larger than 2 cm, the sensitivity increased from 69% to 79%, to 100% reportedly [28].

MDCT is also highly accurate in staging HCC. MDCT can detect the number of lesions, segments involved, regional adenopathy, vascular tumor invasion, and metastases. MDCT also plays a major role in posttreatment evaluation including surveillance following surgical intervention, local therapy, or systemic therapy. For example, in the setting of postablation treatment, follow-up with MDCT may

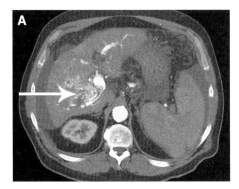
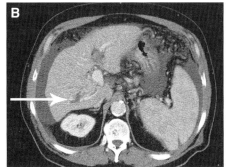

Fig. 16. MDCT evaluation of the abdomen of a 73-year-old man obtained during the late arterial (*A*) and late portal venous phase of enhancement (*B*). There is enhancement of the portal vein during the late arterial phase in keeping with tumor thrombus (*arrow*).

demonstrate a change in enhancement, which is suggestive of tumor recurrence, and in the presurgical patient undergoing portal vein embolization, MDCT is useful in assessing the regeneration of liver parenchyma.

Portal and hepatic vein invasion by HCC may be present. The distinction between tumor thrombus and bland thrombus is aided by the detection of early enhancement of the thrombus during the early or late arterial phase (Fig. 16). The temporal resolution of MDCT permits arterial-only imaging without contamination of portal-venous flow. A pitfall of the faster MDCT examinations is increased incidence of detection of hepatic perfusion abnormalities. It is important to recognize this process to avoid confusion with malignancy (Fig. 17). The etiology of these changes may be caused by anatomic variants, vascular obstruction, and arterioportal shunting.

Recognition of these findings can reduce the number of false-positive diagnoses.

The application of MDCT technology in patients with HCC now permits an increased sensitivity of detection, improved staging, and improved therapeutic planning for percutaneous regional therapy or surgical management.

Cholangiocarcinoma

Cholangiocarcinoma is the second most common primary hepatobiliary malignancy, after HCC. These tumors can be divided into intrahepatic and extrahepatic locations. Tumors at the periphery of the biliary tree are intrahepatic cholangiocarcinoma. Peripheral cholangiocarcinomas are usually large because they are rarely symptomatic early in their course. These account for 10% of cholangiocarcino-

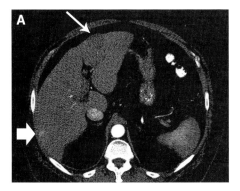
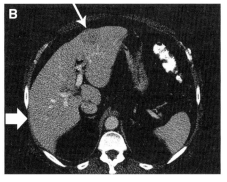

Fig. 17. MDCT evaluation of the abdomen of a 68-year-old man obtained during the late arterial (*A*) and late portal venous phase of enhancement (*B*). There is a hepatoma in the left lobe of the liver (*thin arrow*). There is also a hypervascular, wedge-shaped, peripheral area seen during the earlier phase of enhancement that is isoattenuating to live on delayed images (*thick arrow*). The latter is consistent with perfusion abnormality and not a HCC.

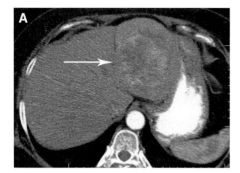 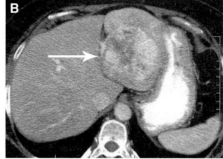

Fig. 18. MDCT evaluation of the abdomen in a 51-year-old woman with intrahepatic cholangiocarcinoma. The images were obtained during the late arterial phase (*A*) and portal venous phase (*B*) of enhancement. There is a mass in the left lobe of the liver that demonstrates rimlike contrast enhancement during the earlier stages of contrast administration and enhances during the portal venous phase of enhancement in keeping with intrahepatic cholangiocarcinomas (*arrow*).

mas and have a distinct clinical presentation, diagnostic imaging findings, and management.

The clinical features of intrahepatic cholangiocarcinomas include right upper quadrant pain, weight loss, hepatomegaly, fever, and weakness. The presence of jaundice is not characteristic of intrahepatic cholangiocarcinoma. This is a feature of the extrahepatic form. The laboratory findings of elevated bilirubin, CA-19 markers, and liver enzymes that are characteristic of extrahepatic cholangiocarcinoma are not seen with intrahepatic cholangiocarcinoma. The tumor staging is the same as for HCC. The tumor (T) classification is based on the numbers of nodules present, the size of nodules, and the presence of vascular invasion.

Grossly, intrahepatic cholangiocarcinomas is a firm hypovascular tumor with predominantly fibrous stroma. Histologically, it is usually a well-differentiated sclerosing adenocarcinoma with abundant desmoplasia. The pathologic evaluation of intrahepatic cholangiocarcinomas is difficult. It is not possible to distinguish intrahepatic cholangiocarcinomas from metastatic carcinoma on morphologic features alone. Such differentiation is typically dependent on the identification of an extrahepatic primary carcinoma in the case of metastatic disease [113].

Treatment options include surgery (resection or transplant); percutaneous regional therapy; and systemic therapy. Of the available therapies, surgery offers the best treatment option. The prognosis of patients with intrahepatic cholangiocarcinomas is poor because many are not detected until an advanced stage, making curative surgery difficult.

Imaging plays an essential role in the clinical management of these patients, with CT and MR imaging as the most commonly used imaging modalities in the diagnosis, staging, and surveillance of the disease.

The most common CT appearance of cholangiocarcinoma is that of a low-attenuation mass with irregular margins with mild peripheral enhancement on the delayed phase of imaging (Fig. 18). This delayed enhancement is a result of slow diffusion of contrast into the interstitial space and results in prolonged enhancement. Satellite nodules, regional lymph nodes, and capsule retraction may be present. Rimlike contrast enhancement is one of the most frequent patterns observed in either arterial- or portal-phase imaging (see Fig. 18) [114].

In contrast to HCC, these tumors usually do not invade adjacent vessels but encase them. Invasion of the bile ducts (Fig. 19), perineural spaces, and lymphatic vessels is seen, however, resulting in lymph node metastasis and intrahepatic metastasis [114,115]. The appearance of cholangiocarcinoma

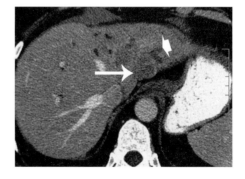

Fig. 19. MDCT evaluation of the abdomen of a 56-year-old woman with intrahepatic cholangiocarcinoma. The images were obtained during the late portal venous phase of enhancement. There is low-attenuation mass with irregular peripheral enhancement (*thin arrow*); there is atrophy of the left lobe, and biliary dilatation (*thick arrow*). The left hepatic vein is not visualized, most likely encased by tumor.

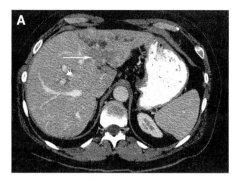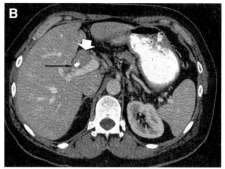

Fig. 20. (*A*) MDCT evaluation of the abdomen of a 56-year-old woman with intrahepatic cholangiocarcinoma. The images were obtained during the late portal venous phase of enhancement. There is a soft tissue attenuation mass in the left lobe of the liver (*arrow*). (*B*) On the lower slice there is a soft tissue mass within the bile duct in keeping with tumor extension (*white arrow*). A bile duct stent is seen (*black arrow*).

during dynamic postcontrast images and during prolonged delayed images has been evaluated. Most tumors are hypoattenuating during the dynamic studies and hyperattenuating during prolonged delayed images (10–20 minutes postcontrast administration) [115,116].

In the proper clinical setting, detection of a hypodense hepatic lesion with peripheral enhancement, biliary dilatation, atrophy, and contrast enhancement on delayed images is highly suggestive of peripheral intrahepatic cholangiocarcinoma (Fig. 20).

Liver metastases

Metastatic spread of tumor to the liver is much more common than the occurrence of primary liver malignancy. The most common tumors to metastasize to the liver are colon, lung, pancreatic, melanoma, and sarcoma [86].

Except for infiltrative tumors, such as lymphoma, most metastatic disease to the liver manifests on CT as multiple masses, usually with ill-defined margins and an irregular rim. Those lesions that enhance rapidly, such as metastatic disease from breast cancer, renal cell carcinoma, thyroid cancer, and neuroendocrine or carcinoid tumors, appear hyperdense compared with normal liver parenchyma particularly on arterial phases of imaging (Fig. 21) and may appear isodense, or hypodense, to the normal liver parenchyma on the portal-venous phase of imaging. In contrast, most metastatic liver disease arising from gastrointestinal tract tumors, such as colon cancer, typically is best identified as hypodense lesions on the portal-venous phase of imaging (Fig. 22).

Most reports on the accuracy of CT for detecting liver lesions are based on experience with single-detector spiral CT. A recent study of dual-phase spiral CT for the detection and characterization of liver lesions (primary and metastatic) showed a sensitivity

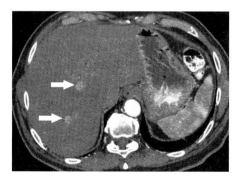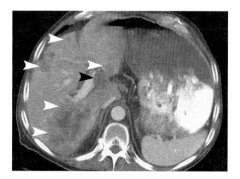

Fig. 21. A 77-year-old-man with history of pancreatic islet cell tumor, with hypervascular liver metastases (*arrows*) seen on arterial phase of multiphase CT study.

Fig. 22. A 61-year-old man with a history of gastric cancer. Multiple liver metastases (*white arrowheads*) and porta hepatitis adenopathy (*black arrowhead*) are present.

of 69% to 71% for malignant disease [117]. Detection rate seems to vary with regard to the primary tumor type and the nature of hepatic metastatic disease (intraparenchymal or peritoneal). The sensitivity for detecting colon cancer metastases to the liver has been reported to be 85% [118]. In contrast, one of the few studies using thin-section MDCT, and multiplanar reformatted images, showed that the detection rate for peritoneal implants for ovarian cancer to the liver surface and diaphragm, including small implants and miliary disease, was approximately 50% [119]. One of the difficulties in identifying metastatic disease is the high incidence of small (<15 mm) benign lesions that appear indeterminate on CT. A study of 209 patients with a known primary tumor showed that 51% of lesions identified that were <15 mm in diameter were benign [120]. Close follow-up is often advised to monitor for the development of liver metastases and to characterize small lesions.

Summary

MDCT scanners with subsecond gantry rotation times provide several advantages including faster scan time, increased scan range, and thinner collimation with improved z-axis resolution. Better definition of different phases of hepatic enhancement and shorter scanning times have increased the importance of scan timing and have led to re-evaluation and modification of existing CT protocols and contrast administration strategies. The newest scanners permit high-quality three-dimensional imaging of the liver and optimize MPR and three-dimensional reconstructions. MDCT technology improves the capability of CT to detect and characterize focal liver lesions and also expands its indications by allowing three-dimensional display of vascular and parenchymal structures.

References

[1] Bryant T, Blomley M, Albrecht T, et al. Improved characterization of liver lesions with liver-phase uptake of liver-specific microbubbles: prospective multicenter study. Radiology 2004;232:799–809.

[2] Lee V, Lavelle M, Rofsky N, et al. Hepatic MR imaging with a dynamic contrast-enhanced isotropic volumetric interpolated breath-hold examination: feasibility, reproducibility, and technical quality. Radiology 2000;215:365–72.

[3] Sahani D, Saini S, Pena C, et al. Using multidetector CT for preoperative vascular evaluation of liver neoplasms: technique and results. AJR Am J Roentgenol Am J Roentgenol 2002;179:53–9.

[4] Sahani D, Krishnamurthy S, Kalva S, et al. Multidetector-row computed tomography angiography for planning intra-arterial chemotherapy pump placement in patients with colorectal metastases to the liver. J Comput Assist Tomogr 2004;28: 478–84.

[5] Guiney MJ, Kruskal JB, Sosna J, et al. Multi-detector row CT of relevant vascular anatomy of the surgical plane in split-liver transplantation. Radiology 2003; 229:401–7.

[6] Schroeder T, Nadalin S, Stattaus J, et al. Potential living liver donors: evaluation with an all-in-one protocol with multi-detector row CT. Radiology 2002;224:586–91.

[7] Hu H, He DH, Foley DW, et al. Four multidetector-row helical CT: image quality and volume coverage speed. Radiology 2000;215:55–62.

[8] Spielmann AL, Nelson RC, Lowry CR, et al. Liver: single breath-hold dynamic subtraction CT with multidetector row helical technology feasibility study. Radiology 2002;222:278–83.

[9] Nakashige A, Horiguchi J, Tamura A, et al. Quantitative measurement of hepatic portal perfusion by multidetector row CT with compensation for respiratory misregistration. Br J Radiol 2004;77: 728–34.

[10] Tsushima Y, Funabasama S, Aoki J, et al. Quantitative perfusion map of malignant liver tumors, created for dynamic computed tomography data. Acad Radiol 2004;11:215–23.

[11] Weg N, Scheer MR, Gabor MP. Liver lesions: improved detection with dual-detector-array CT and routine 2.5-mm thin collimation. Radiology 1998; 209:417–26.

[12] Haider MA, Amitai MM, Rappaport DC, et al. Multi-detector row helical CT in preoperative assessment of small (≤1.5cm) liver metastases: is thinner collimation better? Radiology 2002;225:137–42.

[13] Kawata S, Murakami T, Kim T, et al. Multidetector CT: diagnostic impact of slice thickness on detection of hypervascular hepatocellular carcinoma. AJR Am J Roentgenol 2002;179:61–6.

[14] Brancatelli G, Federle MP, Katyal S, et al. Hemodynamic characterization of focal nodular hyperplasia using three-dimensional volume-rendered multidetector CT angiography. AJR Am J Roentgenol 2002;179: 81–5.

[15] Kamel IR, Georgiades C, Fishman EK. Incremental value of advanced image processing of multislice computed tomography data in the evaluation of hypervascular liver lesions. J Comput Assist Tomogr 2003;27:652–6.

[16] Kamel IR, Lawler L, Fishman EK. Comprehensive analysis of hypervascular liver lesions using 16-MDCT and advanced image processing. AJR Am J Roentgenol 2004;183:443–52.

[17] Stemmler BJ, Paulson EK, Thornton FJ, et al. Dual-Phase three-dimensional MDCT angiography for evaluation of the liver before hepatic resection. AJR Am J Roentgenol 2004;183:1551–7.

[18] Kang HK, Jeong YY, Choi JH, et al. Three-dimensional multi-detector row CT portal venography in the evaluation of portosystemic collateral vessels in liver cirrhosis. Radiographics 2002;22:1053–61.

[19] Tanikake M, Shimizu T, Narabayashi I, et al. Three-dimensional CT angiography of the hepatic artery: use of multi-detector row helical CT and a contrast agent. Radiology 2003;227:883–9.

[20] Onodera Y, Omatsu T, Nakayama J, et al. Peripheral anatomic evaluation using three-dimensional CT hepatic venography in donors: significance of peripheral venous visualization in living-donor liver transplantation. AJR Am J Roentgenol 2004;183:1065–70.

[21] Lee SS, Kim TK, Byun JH, et al. Hepatic arteries in potential donors for living related liver transplantation: evaluation with multi-detector row CT angiography. Radiology 2003;227:391–9.

[22] Lang H, Radtke A, Liu C, et al. Extended left hepatectomy: modified operation planning based on three-dimensional visualization of liver anatomy. Langenbecks Arch Surg 2004;389:306–10.

[23] Wigmore SJ, Redhead DN, Yan XJ, et al. Virtual hepatic resection using three-dimensional reconstruction of helical computed tomography angioportograms. Ann Surg 2001;233:221–6.

[24] Foley DW, Mallisee TA, Hohenwalter MD, et al. Multiphase hepatic CT with a multirow detector CT scanner. AJR Am J Roentgenol 2000;175:679–85.

[25] Murakami T, Kim T, Takamura M, et al. Hypervascular hepatocellular carcinoma: detection with double arterial phase multi-detector row helical CT. Radiology 2001;218:763–7.

[26] Kim SK, Lim JH, Lee WJ, et al. Detection of hepatocellular carcinoma: comparison of dynamic three-phase computed tomography images and four-phase computed tomography images using multi-detector row helical computed tomography. J Comput Assist Tomogr 2002;26:691–8.

[27] Ichikawa T, Kitamura T, Nakajima H, et al. Hypervascular hepatocellular carcinoma: can double arterial phase imaging with multidetector CT improve tumor depiction in the cirrhotic liver? AJR Am J Roentgenol 2002;179:751–8.

[28] Laghi A, Iannaccone R, Rossi P, et al. Hepatocellular carcinoma: detection with triple-phase multi-detector row helical CT in patients with chronic hepatitis. Radiology 2003;226:543–9.

[29] Francis IR, Cohan RH, McNulty NJ, et al. Multidetector CT of the liver and hepatic neoplasms: effect of multiphasic imaging on tumor conspicuity and vascular enhancement. AJR Am J Roentgenol 2003;180:1217–24.

[30] Lim JH, Choi D, Kim SH, et al. Detection of hepatocellular carcinoma: value of adding delayed phase imaging to dual-phase helical CT. AJR Am J Roentgenol 2002;179:67–73.

[31] Keogan MT, Seabourn JT, Paulson EK, et al. Contrast-enhanced CT of intrahepatic and hilar cholangiocarcinoma: delay time for optimal imaging. AJR Am J Roentgenol 1997;169:1493–9.

[32] Lee TY, Purdie TG, Stewart E. CT imaging of angiogenesis. Q J Nucl Med 2003;47:171–87.

[33] Brink JA, Wang G, McFarland EG. Optimal section spacing in single-detector helical CT. Radiology 2000;214:575–8.

[34] Urban BA, Fishman EK, Kuhlman JE, et al. Detection of focal hepatic lesions with spiral CT: comparison of 4- and 8-mm interscan spacing. AJR Am J Roentgenol 1993;160:783–5.

[35] Saini S. Multi-detector row CT: principles and practice for abdominal applications. Radiology 2004;233:323–7.

[36] Silverman P, Kalender W, Hazle J. Common terminology for single and multislice helical CT. AJR Am J Roentgenol 2001;176:1135–6.

[37] Nelson R, Spielmann A. Liver imaging with multidetector helical computed tomography. J Comput Assist Tomogr 2003;27(Suppl 1):S9–16.

[38] Brink J. Use of high concentration contrast media (HCCM): principles and rationale—body CT. Eur J Radiol 2003;45(Suppl 1):S53–8.

[39] Awai K, Takada K, Onishi H, et al. Aortic and hepatic enhancement and tumor-to-liver contrast: analysis of the effect of different concentrations of contrast material at multi-detector row helical CT. Radiology 2002;224:757–63.

[40] Furuta A, Ito K, Fujita T, et al. Hepatic enhancement in multiphasic contrast-enhanced MDCT: comparison of high- and low-iodine-concentration contrast med in same patients with chronic liver disease. AJR Am J Roentgenol 2004;183:157–62.

[41] Bae KT. Peak contrast enhancement in CT and MR angiography: when does it occur and why? Pharmacokinetic study in a porcine model. Radiology 2003;227:809–16.

[42] Brink JA. Contrast optimization and scan timing for single and multidetector-row computed tomography. J Comput Assist Tomogr 2003;27(Suppl 1):S3–8.

[43] Hopper KD, Mosher TJ, Kasales CJ, et al. Thoracic spiral CT: delivery of contrast material pushed with injectable saline solution in a power injector. Radiology 1997;205:269–71.

[44] Dorio PJ, Lee Jr FT, Henseler KP, et al. Using a saline chaser to decrease contrast media in abdominal CT. AJR Am J Roentgenol 2003;180:929–34.

[45] Schoellnast H, Tillich M, Deutschmann HA, et al. Abdominal multidetector row computed tomography: reduction of cost and contrast material dose using saline flush. J Comput Assist Tomogr 2003;27:847–53.

[46] Heiken JP, Brink JA, McClennan BL, et al. Dynamic incremental CT: effect of volume and concentration of contrast material and patient weight on hepatic enhancement. Radiology 1995;195:353–7.

[47] Bae KT, Heiken JP, Brink JA. Aortic hepatic contrast medium enhancement at CT. Part II: Effect of reduced cardiac output in a porcine model. Radiology 1998; 207:657–62.

[48] Kim T, Murakami T, Hori M, et al. Small hypervascular hepatocellular carcinoma revealed by double arterial phase CT performed with single breath-hold scanning and automatic bolus tracking. AJR Am J Roentgenol 2002;178:899–904.

[49] Itoh S, Ikeda M, Achiwa M, et al. Late-arterial and portal-venous phase imaging of the liver with multislice CT scanner in patients without circulatory disturbances: automatic bolus tracking or empirical scan delay? Eur Radiol 2004;14:1665–73.

[50] Yoshizumi TT, Nelson RC. Radiation issues with multidetector row helical CT. Computed Tomography 2003;44:95–117.

[51] Kalra MK, Maher MM, Toth TL, et al. Strategies for CT radiation dose optimization. Radiology 2004;230: 619–28.

[52] Carrim ZI, Murchison JT. The prevalence of simple renal and hepatic cysts detected by spiral computed tomography. Clin Radiol 2003;58:626–9.

[53] Inaba T, Nagashima I, Ogawa F, et al. Diffuse intrahepatic bile duct dilation caused by a very small hepatic cyst. J Hepatobiliary Pancreat Surg 2003;10: 106–8.

[54] Zonios D, Soula M, Archimandritis AJ, et al. Cystlike hepatic metastases from gastrointestinal stromal tumors could be seen before any treatment. AJR Am J Roentgenol 2003;181:282.

[55] Chen MY, Bechtold RE, Savage PD. Cystic changes in hepatic metastases from gastrointestinal stromal tumors (GISTs) treated with Gleevec (imatinib mesylate). AJR Am J Roentgenol 2002;179:1059–62.

[56] Halvorsen RA, Korobkin M, Foster WL, et al. The variable CT appearance of hepatic abscesses. AJR Am J Roentgenol 1984;142:941–6.

[57] Mortele KJ, Segatto E, Ros PR. The infected liver: radiologic-pathologic correlation. Radiographics 2004;24:937–55.

[58] Mortele KJ, Ros PR. Cystic focal liver lesions in the adult: differential CT and MR imaging features. Radiographics 2001;21:895–910.

[59] Karhunen PJ. Benign hepatic tumours and tumour like conditions in men. J Clin Pathol 1986;39:183–8.

[60] Leslie DF, Johnson CD, Johnson CM, et al. Distinction between cavernous hemangiomas of the liver and hepatic metastases on CT: value of contrast enhancement patterns. AJR Am J Roentgenol 1995; 164:625–9.

[61] Jang HJ, Kim TK, Lim HK, et al. Hepatic hemangioma: atypical appearances on CT, MR imaging, and sonography. AJR Am J Roentgenol 2003;180: 135–41.

[62] Kim KW, Kim TK, Han JK, et al. Hepatic hemangiomas with arterioportal shunt: findings at two-phase CT. Radiology 2001;219:707–11.

[63] Buetow PC, Pantongrag-Brown L, Buck JL, et al.

[64] Nguyen BN, Flejou JF, Terris B, et al. Focal nodular hyperplasia of the liver: a comprehensive pathologic study of 305 lesions and recognition of new histologic forms. Am J Surg Pathol 1999;23: 1441–54.

[65] Shamsi K, De Schepper A, Degryse H, et al. Focal nodular hyperplasia of the liver: radiologic findings. Abdom Imaging 1993;18:32–8.

[66] Choi CS, Freeny PC. Triphasic helical CT of hepatic focal nodular hyperplasia: incidence of atypical findings. AJR Am J Roentgenol 1998;170:391–5.

[67] Mergo PJ, Ros PR. Benign lesions of the liver. Radiol Clin North Am 1998;36:319–31.

[68] Rooks JB, Ory HW, Ishak KG, et al. Epidemiology of hepatocellular adenoma, the role of oral contraceptive use. JAMA 1979;242:644–8.

[69] Soe KL, Soe M, Gluud S. Liver pathology associated with the use of anabolic-androgenic steroids. Liver Transpl 1992;12:73–9.

[70] Mathieu D, Bruneton JN, Drouillard J, et al. Hepatic adenomas and focal nodular hyperplasia: dynamic CT study. Radiology 1986;160:53–8.

[71] Ichikawa T, Federle MP, Grazioli L, et al. Hepatocellular adenoma: multiphasic CT and histopathologic findings in 25 patients. Radiology 2000;214:861–8.

[72] Ito K, Honjo K, Fujita T, et al. Liver neoplasms: diagnostic pitfalls in cross-sectional imaging. Radiographics 1996;16:273–93.

[73] Flowers BF, McBurney RP, Vera SR. Ruptured hepatic adenoma: a spectrum of presentation and treatment. Am Surg 1990;56:380–3.

[74] Gordon SC, Reddy KR, Livingston AS. Resolution of a contraceptive steroid induced hepatic adenoma with subsequent evolution into HCC. Ann Intern Med 1986;105:547–9.

[75] Kubota E, Katsumi K, Iida M, et al. Biliary cystadenocarcinoma followed up as benign cystadenoma for 10 years. J Gastroenterol 2003;38:278–82.

[76] Matsuoka Y, Hayashi K, Yano M, et al. Case report: malignant transformation of biliary cystadenoma with mesenchymal stroma: documentation by CT. Clin Radiol 1997;52:318–21.

[77] Devaney K, Goodman ZD, Ishak KG. Hepatobiliary cystadenoma and cystadenocarcinoma: a light microscopic and immunohistochemical study of 70 patients. Am J Surg Pathol 1994;18:1078–91.

[78] Buetow PC, Buck JL, Pantongrag-Brown L, et al. Biliary cystadenoma and cystadenocarcinoma: clinical-imaging-pathologic correlation with emphasis on the importance of ovarian stroma. Radiology 1995; 196:805–10.

[79] Korobkin M, Stephens DH, Lee JK, et al. Biliary cystadenoma and cystadenocarcinoma: CT and sonographic findings. AJR Am J Roentgenol 1989;153: 507–11.

[80] Hara H, Morita S, Sako S, et al. Hepatobiliary

cystadenoma combined with multiple liver cysts: report of a case. Surg Today 2001;31:651–4.

[81] Florman SS, Slakey DP. Giant biliary cystadenoma: case report and literature review. Am Surg 2001;67: 727–32.

[82] Land MA, Moinuddin M, Bisno AL. Pyogenic liver abscess: changing epidemiology and prognosis. South Med J 1985;78:1426–30.

[83] Mathieu D, Vasile N, Fagniez PL, et al. Dynamic CT features of hepatic abscesses. Radiology 1985;154: 749–52.

[84] Jeffrey Jr RB, Tolentino CS, Chang FC, et al. CT of small pyogenic hepatic abscesses: the cluster sign. AJR Am J Roentgenol 1988;151:487–9.

[85] Terrier F, Becker CD, Triller JK. Morphologic aspects of hepatic abscesses at computed tomography and ultrasound. Acta Radiol Diagn (Stockh) 1983;24: 129–37.

[86] Bluemke DA, Soyer P, Fishman EK. Helical (spiral) CT of the liver. Radiol Clin North Am 1995;33:863–86.

[87] Ralls PW. Focal inflammatory disease of the liver. Radiol Clin North Am 1998;36:377–89.

[88] Radin DR, Ralls PW, Colletti PM, et al. CT of amebic liver abscess. AJR Am J Roentgenol 1988;150: 1297–301.

[89] Hollett MD, Jeffrey Jr RB, Nino-Murcia M, et al. Dual-phase helical CT of the liver: value of arterial phase scans in the detection of small (1.5cm) malignant hepatic neoplasms. AJR Am J Roentgenol 1995;164:879–84.

[90] Valls C, Cos M, Figueras J, et al. Pretransplantation diagnosis and staging of hepatocellular carcinoma in patients with cirrhosis: value of dual-phase helical CT. AJR Am J Roentgenol 2004;182:1011–7.

[91] Lim JH, Park CK. Hepatocellular carcinoma in advanced liver cirrhosis: CT detection in transplant patients. Abdom Imaging 2004;29:203–7.

[92] Van Thiel DH, Yong S, Li SD, et al. The development of de novo hepatocellular carcinoma in patients on a liver transplant list: frequency, size, and assessment of current screening methods. Liver Transpl 2004;10: 631–7.

[93] Shaked A, McDiarmid S, Harrison R, et al. Hepatic artery thrombosis resulting in gas gangrene of the transplanted liver. Surgery 1992;4:462–5.

[94] Heestand G, Sher L, Lightfoote J, et al. Characteristics and management of splenic artery aneurysm in liver transplant candidates and recipients. Am Surg 2003;69:933–40.

[95] Nghiem HV. Imaging of hepatic transplantation. Radiol Clin North Am 1998;36:429–43.

[96] Yeh BM, Breiman RS, Taouli B, et al. Biliary tract depiction in living potential liver donors: comparison of conventional MR, mangafodipir trisodium-enhanced excretory MR, and multi-detector row CT cholangiography—initial experience. Radiology 2004;230:645–51.

[97] Kamel IR, Lawler LP, Fishman EK. Variations in anatomy of the middle hepatic vein and their impact on formal right hepatectomy. Abdom Imaging 2003; 28:668–74.

[98] Hiroshige S, Shimada M, Harada N, et al. Accurate preoperative estimation of liver-graft volumetry using three-dimensional computed tomography. Transplantation 2003;75:1561–4.

[99] Said A, Safdar N, Lucey MR, et al. Infected bilomas in liver transplant recipients, incidence, risk factors and implications for prevention. Am J Transplant 2004;4:574–82.

[100] Brancatelli G, Katyal S, Federle MP, et al. Three-dimensional multislice helical computed tomography with the volume rendering technique in the detection of vascular complications after liver transplantation. Transplantation 2002;73:237–42.

[101] Katyal S, Oliver III JH, Buck DG, et al. Detection of vascular complications after liver transplantation: early experience in multislice CT angiography with volume rendering. AJR Am J Roentgenol 2000;175: 1735–9.

[102] Moody A, Wilson S, Greig P. Non-Hodgkin lymphoma in the porta hepatis after orthotopic liver transplantation: sonographic findings. Radiology 1992;169:417–20.

[103] Boraschi P, Donati F. Complications of orthotopic liver transplantation: imaging findings. Abdom Imaging 2004;29:189–202.

[104] Mergo PJ, Ros PR. Imaging of diffuse liver disease. Radiol Clin North Am 1998;36:365–75.

[105] McKusick MA. Imaging findings in Budd-Chiari syndrome. Liver Transpl 2001;7:743–4.

[106] Giovine S, Romano L, Aragiusto G, et al. Budd-Chiari syndrome: retrospective study of 8 cases assessed with computerized tomography. Radiol Med (Torino) 1998;96:339–43.

[107] Bradbury MS, Kavanagh PV, Chen MY, et al. Noninvasive assessment of portomesenteric venous thrombosis: current concepts and imaging strategies. J Comput Assist Tomogr 2002;26:392–404.

[108] Chae EJ, Goo HW, Kim SC, et al. Congenital intrahepatic arterioportal and portosystemic venous fistulae with jejunal arteriovenous malformation depicted on multislice spiral CT. Pediatr Radiol 2004; 34:428–31.

[109] Vauthey JN, Lauwers GY, Esnaola NF, et al. Simplified staging for hepatocellular carcinoma. J Clin Oncol 2002;20:1527–36.

[110] Pawarode A, Lauwers GY, Esnaola NF, et al. Natural history of untreated primary hepatocellular carcinoma: a retrospective study of 157 patients. Am J Clin Oncol 1998;21:386–91.

[111] Baron RL, Oliver III JH, Dodd III GD, et al. Hepatocellular carcinoma: evaluation with biphasic, contrast-enhanced, helical CT. Radiology 1996;199: 505–11.

[112] Oliver III JH, Baron RL, Federle MP, et al. Detecting hepatocellular carcinoma: value of unenhanced or arterial phase CT imaging or both used in conjunction with conventional portal venous phase contrast-

enhanced CT imaging. AJR Am J Roentgenol 1996; 167:71–7.

[113] Sampatanukul P, Leong AS, Kosolbhand P, et al. Proliferating ductules are a diagnostic discriminator for intrahepatic cholangiocarcinoma in FNA biopsies. Diagn Cytopathol 2000;22:359–63.

[114] Valls C, Guma A, Puig I, et al. Intrahepatic peripheral cholangiocarcinoma: CT evaluation. Abdom Imaging 2000;25:490–6.

[115] Keogan MT, Seabourn JT, Paulson EK, et al. Contrast-enhanced CT of intrahepatic and hilar cholangiocarcinoma: delay time for optimal imaging. AJR Am J Roentgenol 1997;169:1493–9.

[116] Lacomis JM, Baron RL, Oliver III JH, et al. Cholangiocarcinoma: delayed CT contrast enhancement patterns. Radiology 1997;203:98–104.

[117] Kamel IR, Choti MA, Horton KM, et al. Surgically staged focal liver lesions: accuracy and reproducibility of dual-phase helical CT for detection and characterization. Radiology 2003;227:752–7.

[118] Valls C, Andia E, Sanchez A, et al. Hepatic metastases from colorectal cancer: preoperative detection and assessment of resectability with helical CT. Radiology 2001;218:55–60.

[119] Pannu HK, Horton KM, Fishman EK. Thin section dual-phase multidetector-row computed tomography detection of peritoneal metastases in gynecologic cancers. J Comput Assist Tomogr 2003;27:333–40.

[120] Jones EC, Chezmar JL, Nelson RC, et al. The frequency and significance of small (less than or equal to 15 mm) hepatic lesions detected by CT. AJR Am J Roentgenol 1992;158:535–9.

ELSEVIER
SAUNDERS

Radiol Clin N Am 43 (2005) 849 – 860

RADIOLOGIC
CLINICS
of North America

Applications of PET in Liver Imaging

Amir H. Khandani, MD, PhD[a],*, Richard L. Wahl, MD[b]

[a]Section of Nuclear Medicine, Department of Radiology, University of North Carolina, CB 7510,
Chapel Hill, NC 27599–7510, USA
[b]Russell H. Morgan Department of Radiology and Radiological Science, The Johns Hopkins University School of Medicine,
Johns Hopkins Hospital, 600 North Wolfe Street, Baltimore, MD 21287, USA

Although PET has been used for several decades in the research setting, its clinical use has grown substantially in the past decade. PET is a quantitative physiologic imaging modality using positron emitters, such as fluorine-18 (^{18}F), oxygen-15 (^{15}O), nitrogen-13 (^{13}N), and carbon-11 (^{11}C). The fact that these nuclides are components of common biologic molecules makes PET particularly suitable visually to capture different biologic pathways; however, the short physical half-life of ^{15}O (2 minutes), ^{13}N (10 minutes), and ^{11}C (20 minutes) limits their use to the centers with an on-site cyclotron. ^{18}F has a physical half-life of 110 minutes and can be synthesized in commercially operating cyclotrons and transported to remote PET facilities. The most commonly used radiotracer is 2-[^{18}F] fluoro-2-deoxy-D-glucose (FDG).

Tumor imaging with FDG is based on the principle of increased glucose metabolism of cancer cells. Like glucose, FDG is taken up by the cancer cells through facilitative glucose transporters (Glut). Gluts are glycoproteins, and so far 12 isoforms have been identified in different organs. Normal hepatocytes express Glut2, Glut9, and Glut10 [1]. Expression of Gluts, predominantly Glut1 and Glut3, is significantly higher in many cancer cells compared with normal cells.

Once in the cell, glucose or FDG is phosphorylated by hexokinase to glucose-6-phospate or FDG-6-phosphate, respectively. Expression of hexokinase and its affinity or functional activity for phosphory-

lation of glucose or FDG is often higher in cancer cells compared with normal cells; hexokinase II is predominantly expressed in cancer cells. Glucose-6-phosphate travels further down the glycolytic or oxidative pathways to be metabolized, in contrast to FDG-6-phosphate, which cannot go further and cannot be metabolized. In normal cells, glucose-6-phospate or FDG-6-phosphate can be dephosphorylated and exit the cells. In many cancer cells, however, expression of glucose-6-phosphatase is often significantly decreased, and glucose-6-phospate or FDG-6-phosphte can get only minimally dephosphorylated and remains in large part within the cell. Because FDG-6-phosphate cannot be metabolized, it is trapped in the cell as a polar metabolite and can be visualized by PET. In normal liver parenchyma, the concentration of glucose-6-phosphatase is high, which causes rapid clearance of FDG from the liver. This may account for the mild intensity of the normal liver on whole-body PET, especially at later imaging times post tracer injection [2]. In fact, in many publications and clinical routine, intensity of the liver has often been used as reference for background uptake.

Metastatic liver lesions

Metastatic disease accounts for most malignant lesions in the liver, outnumbering primary hepatic malignancies by a ratio of 18 to 1 in the Unites States [3]. Often, the presence of liver metastases is the main determinant of survival and guides the therapeutic strategy, particularly in patients with colorectal cancer [4,5].

* Corresponding author.
E-mail address: khandani@med.unc.edu
(A.H. Khandani).

0033-8389/05/$ – see front matter © 2005 Elsevier Inc. All rights reserved.
doi:10.1016/j.rcl.2005.05.008

Zimmerman and coworkers [6] studied expression of Glut1 in hepatic metastases originating from different primaries, and found that Glut1 was overexpressed in hepatic metastases of 3 of 5 lung primaries, 7 of 11 pancreatic primaries, 7 of 9 colon primaries, 2 of 7 breast primaries, 2 of 2 squamous cell primaries, 1 of 3 biliary tract primaries, and none of neuroendocrine primaries that were examined. To the authors' knowledge, expression of other Gluts, such as Glut3 in hepatic metastases, has never been published.

FDG-PET proved to be highly sensitive in detecting hepatic metastases from different primaries. Delbeke and coworkers [7] studied the diagnostic value of FDG-PET in hepatic metastases measuring 1 cm and larger, and detected all 66 metastatic lesions originating from various primaries, such as the colon, pancreas, esophagus, sarcoma, and parotid. Similar results with overall greater sensitivity of PET compared with spiral CT have been reported by other groups, particularly if CT findings are indeterminate [8–10]. In cases of known solitary hepatic metastasis diagnosed by CT, several groups reported discovery of additional hepatic metastases by FDG-PET [11–13]. This is of particular importance in preoperative evaluation of solitary hepatic metastasis because detection of additional lesions often changes the management. Retrospective data by Fernandez and coworkers [14] has shown that the use of FDG-PET in assessing patients considered for partial hepatectomy for colon cancer liver metastases is associated with superior long-term survival than is seen in patients selected for surgery using standard anatomic imaging methods only, presumably by selecting, with PET, those patients who do not have extrahepatic metastases, and who benefit most from partial hepatectomy. Additionally, in the case of suspected recurrent colorectal cancer, FDG-PET is more sensitive than CT for discovering hepatic metastases with

the potential of detecting disease earlier than CT, so that metastatic disease is more amenable to curative resection [13,15]. Especially, FDG-PET should be considered in the setting of increasing carcinoembryonic antigen (CEA) to assess for hepatic metastases because it has proved to be more sensitive than CT for this purpose [15].

Yang and coworkers [16] reviewed PET and MR imaging studies of 30 patients with histopathologically proved (N = 27) or clinically suspected (N = 3) hepatic metastases from nonhepatic primaries. The sensitivity, specificity, and positive and negative predictive values on MR imaging were 85.7%, 100%, 100%, and 89%, respectively, compared with 71%, 93.7%, 90.9%, and 79% on PET. The difference between the two methods was not statistically significant. Bohm and coworkers [8] demonstrated similar results. In the authors' experience, PET is of particular benefit in case of indeterminate MR imaging findings (Fig. 1).

A meta-analysis of the literature on detection of hepatic metastases from colorectal, gastric, and esophageal cancers by ultrasound, CT, MR imaging, and PET found that in studies with a specificity higher than 85%, the mean weighted sensitivity was 55% (95% CI: 41–68) for ultrasound; 72% (95% CI: 63–80) for CT; 76% (95% CI: 57–91) for MR imaging; and 90% (95% CI: 80–97) for PET. Results of pairwise comparison between imaging modalities demonstrated a greater sensitivity of PET than ultrasound (P = .001); CT (P = .017); and MR imaging (P = .055). The conclusion was that at equivalent specificity, PET is the most sensitive noninvasive imaging modality for the diagnosis of hepatic metastases from colorectal, gastric, and esophageal cancers [17]. CT can be read to achieve a higher sensitivity, but it is at the expense of specificity, because many CT-positive lesions are false-positive. This was shown in a study by Marom and coworkers [18] in

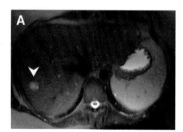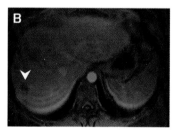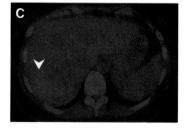

Fig. 1. Patient status post–left hemicolectomy for colon cancer without change in CEA level. MR imaging indicated a lesion in segment VII of the liver with high signal on T2 (*A, arrowhead*) and minimal peripheral enhancement on contrast images (*B, arrowhead*), more characteristic for an atypical hemangioma than metastasis. (*C*) PET was requested to narrow down the differential diagnosis, and indicated intense focal uptake (*arrowhead*). Subsequent biopsy indicated metastatic mucinous adenocarcinoma consistent with colonic primary.

metastatic lung cancer, where in a prospective study of 100 patients nearly twice as many lesions in the liver were identified by CT than by PET; however, all of the incremental lesions identified by CT were false-positives.

False-negative PET for hepatic metastases caused by lower image resolution of PET compared with spiral CT and MR imaging has been reported [8,10,19,20]. It should be considered, however, that these publications were based on non–attenuation-corrected images, which may have lower sensitivity, especially deeper in the abdomen because the deeper areas of the abdomen generally appear much fainter on non–attenuation-corrected than on attenuation-correct PET images. Generally, the role of PET in detecting subcentimeter lesions should be redefined, considering the sophisticated image correction and reconstruction algorithms and higher image resolution of current PET machines. Nonetheless, detection is limited by the sensitivity and the resolution of the scanner and the background tissue radioactivity levels in the normal tissue. Further improvements in image resolution from current 1-cm reconstructed resolution to a few millimeters can be expected with development of small surface area crystal elements in combination with alternative position-sensitive photomultiplier tubes, and the implementation of depth of interaction measurements [21,22]. It is still rare for the reconstructed scanner resolution in patient imaging to match the optimal resolution of the scanner, however, because there often are not enough photon events to depict the true resolution of the scanner. At present, the structural resolution of anatomic imaging remains superior to that of PET. Nonetheless, the diagnostic accuracy of PET is generally superior to anatomic imaging because of its physiologic basis for lesion detection. Another approach to increase detectability of liver metastases has been described by Zasadny and Wahl [23] through acquisition of dynamic PET and forming parametric images of the influx constant. This increases the tumor/background signal ratio and potentially may improve detectability of small lesions; however, it requires more time than standard imaging.

False-negative FDG-PET has also been reported caused by underestimation of uptake, mislocalization of foci, and recent completion of chemotherapy [19,24,25]. The latter is likely associated with microscopic remnant disease at the completion of chemotherapy that regrows and increases in volume with subsequent revisualization on PET once chemotherapy has been terminated. No information is available in the literature, however, on the time interval after completion of chemotherapy during which PET can be false-negative. Based on the authors' experience, this time interval is about 4 to 6 weeks.

Underestimation of uptake of malignant lesions causing false-negative findings on PET can occur because of physiologic movements of the liver during emission scan. The liver is an upper abdominal organ that moves with respiratory movement of the diaphragm. Emission scans are acquired over several minutes during which hepatic lesions, especially those at the dome, are in a repetitive craniocaudal pendulous movement. The respiratory excursion of the liver has been estimated at 10 to 25 mm [26,27]. It is conceivable that cranial and caudal portions of small lesions are registered only half of the acquisition time, and their uptake is underestimated, so that they appear less intense than they really are on images. The degree of this underestimation is variable, and particularly in the case of a subcentimeter lesion this may even lead to nonvisualization of the lesion, as it has been reported by Rohren and coworkers [24]. One way to overcome this problem is to increase the target/background count ratio by increasing the acquisition time. This can be done by increasing the acquisition time of the mid- and upper-abdomen emission frames while acquiring the whole-body scan, if this is possible on the PET machine. Another solution is to acquire a second dedicated scan from mid- and upper-abdomen "liver view" consisting of a transmission scan followed by an emission scan with longer acquisition time, once the whole-body scan is completed (Fig. 2). A different approach to solve this problem is respiratory gating, in which case only emission data collected in certain parts of the respiratory cycle are used for image reconstruction, resulting in better visualization of small lesions with the disadvantage of longer acquisition time [22,28].

Changed position of the liver between emission and transmission scan can cause misalignment between these two images, resulting in mislocalization of hepatic lesions. This is especially of concern when transmission CT is acquired during full inspiration and PET scan is acquired during shallow breathing, but should be less of a problem if the transmission CT is performed during shallow breathing. Osman and coworkers [25] assessed lesion mislocalization among 300 patients using CT and germanium-68 (^{68}Ge) for attenuation correction. The patients were allowed to breathe normally during acquisition of CT and ^{68}Ge transmission scans and during emission scan. There was clinically apparent mislocalization of six right liver dome lesions to the right lung base on the CT attenuation-corrected PET images. In these cases, mislocalization was not apparent on non–

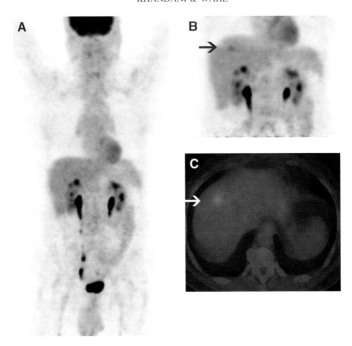

Fig. 2. Patient status post–left hemicolectomy for colon cancer and increasing CEA level. PET was requested for restaging. (*A*) There was no abnormal hepatic focus on the whole-body scan (3 min/frame). (*B* and *C*) The dedicated upper abdomen image "liver view" (6 min/frame) indicted a right hepatic focus (*arrow*). The subsequent segmental resection revealed metastatic adenocarcinoma of colonic primary.

attenuation corrected or ^{68}Ge-attenuation corrected images. Another potential challenge with mislocalization can be caused by foci located below or above the liver, such as those in the hepatic flexure or base of the right lung, to appear to be mislocated "into" the liver [10]. In the authors' experience, this problem is infrequent, but occurs with CT-corrected images and not with longer-duration acquisitions, such as those using ^{68}Ge transmission sources where the duration of image acquisition is similar between the transmission and emission images. In cases of such mislocalizations reviewing the non–attenuation-corrected images is helpful for correct localization of disease.

False-positive findings for malignancy on PET have also been reported caused by intrahepatic abscess; penetrating gallbladder empyema; or benign inflammatory lesions, such as regenerative nodules in a cirrhotic liver [7,8,11].

Given the higher sensitivity of PET in detecting hepatic, and especially extrahepatic, metastasis, it is conceivable that PET will be increasingly used in preoperative staging of malignant tumors. Nonetheless, CT with intravenous contrast or MR imaging is needed for adequate evaluation of anatomic resectability of liver metastases because venous anatomy

in the liver is critical for defining hepatic lobar anatomy. If intravenous-contrast CT is used as an attenuation map, this can produce artifacts with overestimation of FDG uptake in areas of high contrast density; whereas only modest alterations in quantitative PET results do occur if low levels of contrast are present in the blood, high Hounsfield unit attenuation levels can produce rather marked artifacts. In case an intravenous-contrast CT is to be performed, it is recommended to acquire a low- or intermediate-dose unenhanced CT first to be used as an attenuation map, followed by emission scan, after which the intravenous-enhanced CT should be performed. The enhanced CT scan can be performed from the entire body or only from the liver to limit the patient's exposure to radiation [29,30].

3′-[^{18}F]-fluoro-3′-deoxythymidine (FLT) is another PET tracer. Accumulation of FLT in proliferating cells occurs by virtue of the enzyme thymidine kinase I, which is closely linked to the S-phase of cell cycle. This salvage pathway enzyme fluctuates with DNA synthesis, with high activity in proliferating and malignant cells and low or absent activity in quiescent cells [31,32]. Francis and coworkers [31] evaluated the role of FLT in five hepatic metastases from colorectal cancer, and compared FLT uptake with cellular proliferation and FDG uptake. All five lesions were FDG avid. Three of them were also avid for FLT and showed high cellular proliferation (high Ki-67 protein), whereas the remaining two lesions demonstrated no FLT uptake and had very low cellular proliferation. Although FLT-PET has the potential to be used for in vivo grading of malignancy and early prediction of response to chemotherapy, the relatively high physiologic uptake of FLT in the liver makes it a poor candidate for the detection of liver metastases. [methyl-^{11}C] choline also has very intense physiologic hepatic uptake, and is unlikely to be used in the liver imaging.

Hepatocellular carcinoma

HCC or hepatoma develops through malignant transformation of hepatocytes and is common in the setting of chronic liver changes and cirrhosis. HCC is the most common primary epithelial malignancy of the liver, accounting for about 80% of malignant epithelial neoplasms of the liver [33]. HCC has been showing an upward trend in western countries because of the increasing frequency of hepatitis B and C infection [34]. The diagnosis is based on screening risk populations with measurements of serum alpha fetoprotein and liver ultrasound. MR imaging, CT, and lipoidal angiography with follow-up CT are used in inconclusive cases to establish the diagnosis. Biopsy is only performed on patients in whom the radiologic diagnosis cannot be made [35].

Facilitative glucose transporters do not seem to be overexpressed in HCC as often as in other malignant tumors. Zimmerman and coworkers [6] and Roh and coworkers [36] reported expression of Glut1 in 2 of 35 and 1 of 22 examined HCC cases, respectively. Delbeke and coworkers [7] examined a series of 23 patients with HCC. In visual assessment, the tumor/normal liver ratio was definitely high in 13 patients; equivocal (mildly increased compared with normal liver) in three patients; and poor (same or less than the normal liver) in seven patients. The sensitivity of FDG-PET for HCC is about 50% [7,37,38]. There seems to be some association between histologic differentiation of HCC and FDG uptake, with poorly differentiated tumors being more intense on FDG-PET, likely explained by enzymology of HCC. Concentration of glucose-6-phospatase is high in normal liver, causing rapid clearance of glucose-6-phospate or FDG-6-phosphate from hepatocytes with consequent mild appearance of liver on PET. The enzymology of well-differentiated HCC resembles that of the normal liver, likely explaining mild FDG uptake or nonvisualization of these tumors on PET. Less differentiated HCC tumors have lower levels of glucose-6-phosphatase and higher levels of hexokinase, likely causing intense FDG uptake of these tumors on PET [2,39–41]. There seems to be some association between FDG uptake and tumor-volume doubling time and between FDG uptake and tumor size. In a series of 14 HCC tumors, Trojan and coworkers [39] visualized all six HCC tumors larger than 5 cm. FDG-PET could possibly be used to assess the effect of treatment in larger and less differentiated HCC. Shiomi and coworkers [42] and Kong and coworkers [43] demonstrated the usefulness of FDG-PET in predicting the outcome in patients with HCC. Recently, high FDG uptake in HCC has been associated with overexpression of mRNA levels for several markers of aggressive tumor behavior, such as vascular endothelial growth factor [44].

Detection of extrahepatic FDG avid metastases originating from HCC has been reported. Especially in cases of less-differentiated HCC, metastases seem to be more FDG avid [2,39]. Although more data are needed to establish the clinical role of FDG-PET in HCC, in the authors' experience FDG-PET is very helpful to assess the malignant potential of hepatic lesions of unknown primary through simultaneous visualization of the liver and extrahepatic tissue (Fig. 3) and in cases of known HCC with clinically suspected extrahepatic metastasis. Nonetheless, a negative FDG-PET scan in patients with a solitary hepatic lesion does not exclude the possibility of HCC.

[1-^{11}C]-acetate is a short-lived PET tracer with higher uptake in well-differentiated compared with poorly differentiated hepatomas. The physical half-life of ^{11}C acetate is 20 minutes. Several possible pathways of acetate incorporation into tumor metabolism have been postulated; the dominant one seems to be participation in free fatty acid synthesis. Ho and coworkers [2] studied a series of 57 patients with liver lesions, consisting of 39 cases of HCC (group I); 13 cases of non-HCC malignancies (3 cases of cholangiocarcinoma and 10 cases of hepatic metastases from colon, breast, lung, and carcinoid primaries [group II]); and five cases of benign liver lesions (two cases of cavernous hemangioma, two cases of focal nodular hyperplasia, and one case of adenoma [group III]). In group I, there was a complementing sensitivity for HCC on FDG and ^{11}C acetate PET, because these two tracers together gave a sensitivity of 100% for detecting HCC. Most of the well-differentiated HCC lesions were intense on ^{11}C-acetate scan with mild tracer uptake or not visualized on FDG scan, whereas this relationship was reversed for poorly differentiated tumors. In group II,

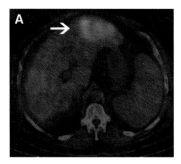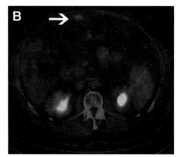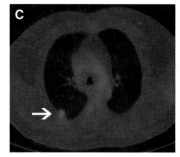

Fig. 3. Patient with left hepatic mass incidentally detected on ultrasound. PET was requested for further assessment, and revealed FDG avidity of the hepatic mass (*A, arrow*) and FDG avid deposits along the anterior abdominal wall (*B, arrow*) and in both lungs, among others in posterior right midlung (*C, arrow*). Image characteristics of the left hepatic mass on MR imaging and alpha fetoprotein level of 897 ng/mL indicated HCC as the primary.

all lesions showed intense FDG uptake but no abnormal ^{11}C-acetate uptake. In group III, the uptake patterns were as follows: hemangiomas were iso-intense on FDG and hypointense on ^{11}C-acetate scan. Both focal nodular hyperplasia cases showed mild intensity uptake on ^{11}C-acetate scan, whereas one of them had mild and another one no visualized uptake on FDG scan. The only adenoma case showed no abnormal FDG or ^{11}C acetate uptake. With an apparently high specificity of ^{11}C-acetate for HCC, the authors concluded that when a lesion is positive for both tracers or only for ^{11}C-acetate, the likelihood of HCC is very high. When a liver lesion is positive only for FDG but is negative for ^{11}C-acetate, the possibility of non-HCC malignancy or poorly differentiated HCC should be considered. In case both tracers are negative, benign pathology is very likely. These conclusions can be particularly helpful for evaluation of tumors <2 cm in patients with low or intermediate likelihood of having HCC (negative serum status for hepatitis B or C, borderline or normal alpha fetoprotein) [2]; however, it must be realized that these very promising data have not been reproduced in a large series and also that the tumors in Asia, where this study was performed, may differ somewhat from the tumors seen in the United States.

Cholangiocarcinoma

Cholangiocarcinoma (CC) originates from the epithelial cells of the biliary tract. After HCC, CC is the second most common primary tumor of the liver, accounting for about 5% to 30% of the primary hepatic malignancies [33]. Biliary obstruction with jaundice is the most common presenting clinical feature in hilar CC, whereas it is uncommon in peripheral CC. The diagnosis of CC has been based on clinical picture, laboratory values, radiologic imaging, and histology, although the latter is often inconclusive in differentiating between CC and metastatic adenocarcinoma. Currently, work-up generally consists of MR imaging, MR cholangiopancreatography, CT, endoscopic retrograde cholangiopancreatography, and percutaneous transhepatic cholangiopancreatography. Overall, the prognosis of this tumor is dismal with 5-year survival as low as 17%; however, improved survival of 22% to 32% at 5 years has been reported with portal or arterial embolization followed by trisegmentectomy [45,46]. Preoperative assessment for hepatic and extrahepatic metastases is likely of prognostic value.

Glut1 is not expressed in normal bile duct, but has been described to be strongly expressed in CC [36,47]. Overall, CC seems to be highly FDG avid and can be visualized on PET if sufficient tumor volume is present. Delbeke and coworkers [7] evaluated eight patients with CC: all lesions demonstrated intense FDG uptake. Hilar and extrahepatic CC, however, have been reported to be less intense on FDG-PET than the peripheral CC, which may be associated with smaller size or higher mucin content of the hilar tumors compared with the peripheral ones [48–50]. Peripheral CC accounts for about 10% of all CC, and often has a characteristic central photopenia on FDG-PET, which corresponds to the central core of fibrotic tissue and desmoplastic reaction provoked by the neoplastic cells; on contrast-enhanced CT or MR imaging, this is evident by early moderate peripheral enhancement followed by progressive and concentric filling [49,51].

FDG-PET is helpful in detecting unsuspected extrahepatic metastatic disease (Fig. 4). Kim and coworkers [49] discovered three unsuspected extra-abdominal lymph nodes and three unsuspected lung metastases in a group of 21 patients with CC. Kato

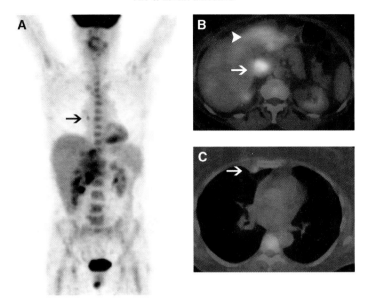

Fig. 4. Patient with poorly differentiated adenocarcinoma of unknown primary diagnosed on a biopsy from a left hepatic lobe mass (*B, arrowhead*). The differential diagnosis included cholangiocarcinoma. PET was requested to stage the patient and evaluate for possible extrahepatic primary. Besides porta hepatis lymph nodes metastases (*B, arrow*), PET revealed a subpleural lesion in the right hemithorax (*A* and *C, arrow*).

and coworkers [48] reported 100% specificity for regional nodal involvement on FDG-PET. Especially in cases of peripheral CC, PET should be considered to evaluate the patient for extrahepatic metastases: peripheral CC attains a large size before it becomes clinically apparent, because it does not obstruct the central biliary system. As a result, extrahepatic metastases are commonly found at the time of diagnosis. In case the histology is inconclusive in differentiating between CC and metastatic adenocarcinoma from extrahepatic primary, FDG-PET should be considered (see Fig. 4).

Gallbladder carcinoma

Gallbladder carcinoma (GBC) is the most common malignant tumor of the biliary tract; this is a highly fatal disease present in 80% to 95% of cases as adenocarcinoma. The diagnosis of GBC is rarely made preoperatively; in most cases GBC presents as an incidental finding at the time of cholecystectomy for presumed benign etiology [52,53].

In postcholecystectomy setting, in patients with T1a (tumor invades mucosa), simple cholecystectomy is regarded as adequate treatment, but these represent only about 16% of all GBC cases [53]. Patients with T1b tumors (tumor invades muscularis)

and beyond should be further evaluated for spread of disease because T1b tumors are associated with lymph node involvement in 15% of cases versus 2.5% of cases with T1a disease [52].

Kim and coworkers [54] examined 71 cases of GBC and demonstrated expression of Glut1 in 37 cases (52.1%). Preoperatively, FDG-PET has been used to distinguish malignant from benign gallbladder lesions with a sensitivity of 75% (six of eight patients), and specificity of 87.5% (seven of eight patients) [55]. Anderson and coworkers [56] used PET to assess possible local residual and metastatic disease after cholecystectomy. PET detected local residual disease in seven (78%) of nine cases, and remote metastases in two of three cases. PET, however, detected only three of six cases with carcinomatosis. In the authors' experience, PET is very helpful to assess for local residual and metastatic disease (Fig. 5).

There has been some concern that nonspecific uptake in the early postsurgical period may disturb image interpretation. Although surgical scars can accumulate FDG for several weeks after the surgical procedure, the pattern of uptake (round and localized for malignancy versus diffuse for inflammation) is often very helpful in distinguishing malignancy from nonspecific postoperative changes. There have been no systematic studies or publications concerning FDG uptake in a postoperative setting. The decision to per-

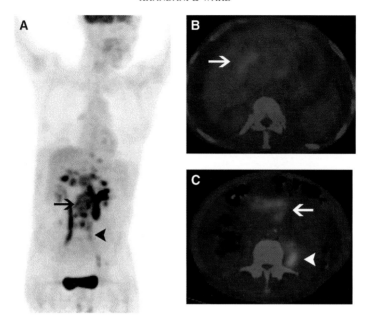

Fig. 5. Patient after laparoscopic cholecystectomy for gallstones was discovered to have moderately differentiated adenocarcinoma of the gallbladder with muscularis invasion. PET was requested for staging, which besides residual local tumor (*B, arrow*) revealed extensive mesenteric (*A* and *C, arrow*) and retroperitoneal (*A* and *C, arrowhead*) lymph node metastases.

form PET to assess for local residual disease should strongly take into account the clinical factors, such as T-stage, and not merely the postoperative time interval.

Monitoring the effect of systemic treatment

FDG-PET has been proved more accurate than CT and MR imaging in assessing the effect of chemotherapy. Effective chemotherapy is associated with a decreased number of tumor cells, and consequently decreased FDG uptake of the tumor mass [57]. FDG-PET can differentiate responders from nonresponders as early as after one to two cycles of chemotherapy with curative approach, such as in lymphoma [58–60], and in neoadjuvant chemotherapy, such as in esophageal and breast cancer [61–63].

In case of hepatic metastases from colon cancer, Findlay and coworkers [64] evaluated the use of FDG-PET in early assessment of chemotherapy. They demonstrated that 4 to 5 weeks after beginning treatment with 5-fluorouracil with or without interferon alpha-2b, the tumor/liver ratio of FDG uptake was significantly lower in responders compared with nonresponders. Although they were not able to discriminate responders from nonresponders after 1 to 2 weeks, this was likely because of technical limitations and low resolution of the equipment used;

in this study, PET scans were acquired on a MUP-PET consisting of two opposed multiwire proportional chambers mounted on a rotating gantry. Dimitrakopoulou-Strauss and coworkers [65] used PET to evaluate the response to chemotherapy with fluorouracil, folinic acid, and oxaliplatin in hepatic metastases. They could predict progressive disease in 96% of the cases. Recently, Goerres and coworkers [66] studied 34 patients with gastrointestinal stromal tumors, 16 of them with liver metastases. They demonstrated that patients without FDG uptake after the start of treatment had a better prognosis than patients with residual uptake. In practice, FDG uptake in the liver is used to monitor treatment response of hepatic lesions with the expectation that such tumors are very likely to behave in a similar manner as do tumor metastases in other locations in the body.

Detecting residual disease after local treatment

For selective treatment of liver tumors, such techniques as radiofrequency ablation, cryosurgery ablation, transcatheter chemoembolization, and arterial chemotherapy infusion have been increasingly used. Despite improvements, these techniques are hampered by limitations in monitoring the effect of treatment. Because the rate of residual disease in tumors

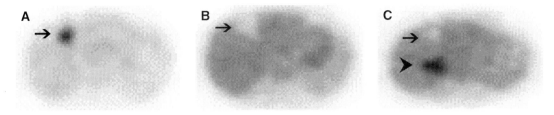

Fig. 6. (*A*) Patient with metastasis from colonic primary in the anterior right hepatic lobe (*arrow*). (*B*) Eight days after radiofrequency ablation, PET indicated photopenia in that location without evidence for residual uptake consistent with complete ablation (*arrow*). (*C*) Three months later, PET revealed a new metastasis in the posterior right hepatic lobe (*arrowhead*); in the anterior right hepatic lobe, there was still complete photopenia (*arrow*), confirming the correct assessment of successful treatment by PET at 8 days.

larger than 3 cm seems to be as high as 48%, short-term follow-up and repeat of the local ablation is of great benefit. Incomplete ablation caused by close vicinity of the tumor to major vessels and resulting so-called "heat-sink" effect has been reported [67,68].

In the first month after radiofrequency ablation, the ability of CT and MR imaging to assess for residual tumor is limited because of the presence of ablation-induced necrosis, edema, and hyperemia in and around the ablated lesion. Conventionally, CT or MR imaging at 1 month is performed to assess for residual tumor [67,68]. There has been increasing evidence that PET is capable of detecting residual tumor earlier than CT and MR imaging (Fig. 6). It has been documented that PET is capable of visualizing residual disease as soon as 7 days after radiofrequency ablation. Donckier and coworkers [69] compared PET with CT in 28 metastatic liver lesions 1 week, 1 month, and 3 months after radiofrequency ablation. In all 28 lesions, CT scans at 1 week, 1 month, and 3 months revealed large nonenhancing regions at the sites of ablation without indication of residual tumor. PET performed 1 week after radiofrequency ablation, however, detected residual disease in four lesion, which was confirmed by histology (N = 3) or CT at 6 months (N = 1). In the remaining 24 lesions, complete ablation was visualized on PET at 1 week as total photopenia, which was subsequently confirmed on follow-up CT or PET with a median follow-up time of 11 months. This is based on the simple fact that cell death is followed by immediate decrease of FDG uptake of the tumor mass on PET. FDG-PET has also been shown to be useful and more accurate than conventional imaging modalities in demonstrating the effect of other local treatments, such as cryosurgery ablation, transcatheter arterial chemoembolization, Y-90 glass microsphere treatment, and microwave coagulation therapy in primary and metastatic malignant liver lesions [70–75].

Protein synthesis rate of the liver

Ishiwata and coworkers [76] measured the protein synthesis rate of the liver in mice using ^{11}C tyrosine. This agent has the potential to be used for assessment of liver function after transplant; currently, there are no reliable methods available for this purpose.

Summary

FDG-PET imaging has an important role in determining if there are metastases to the liver and whether disease has spread beyond the liver. Such information is critical for planning surgical resections of liver metastases. Although FDG-PET can fail to detect many HCCs, it does detect many of the poorly differentiated ones and other PET tracers are showing promise for the detection of better-differentiated hepatomas. Although low-volume CC can escape detection by FDG-PET, higher-volume lesions are well detectable. Similarly, GBC is generally well detected by FDG-PET. The ability of FDG-PET quantitatively to estimate metabolic rates makes it an important tool for monitoring. With increasingly broad indications for FDG-PET imaging, it is expected that FDG-PET (and PET-CT) of the liver will play a growing and increasingly important role in detecting and monitoring treatment of tumors involving the liver.

References

[1] Joost HG, Thorens B. The extended GLUT-family of sugar/polyol transport facilitators: nomenclature, sequence characteristics, and potential function of its novel members. Mol Membr Biol 2001;18:247–56.

[2] Ho CL, Yu SC, Yeung DW. 11C-acetate PET imaging in hepatocellular carcinoma and other liver masses. J Nucl Med 2003;44:213–21.

[3] Brant WE. Liver. In: Webb WR, Brant WE, Helms CA, editors. Fundamentals of body CT. 2nd edition. Philadelphia: WB Saunders; 1998. p. 195–212.

[4] Goslin R, Steele Jr G, Zamcheck N, et al. Factors influencing survival in patients with hepatic metastases from adenocarcinoma of the colon or rectum. Dis Colon Rectum 1982;25:749–54.

[5] Steele Jr G, Ravikumar TS. Resection of hepatic metastases from colorectal cancer: biologic perspective. Ann Surg 1989;210:127–38.

[6] Zimmerman RL, Burke M, Young NA, et al. Diagnostic utility of Glut-1 and CA 15–3 in discriminating adenocarcinoma from hepatocellular carcinoma in liver tumors biopsied by fine-needle aspiration. Cancer 2002;96:53–7.

[7] Delbeke D, Martin WH, Sandler MP, et al. Evaluation of benign vs malignant hepatic lesions with positron emission tomography. Arch Surg 1998;133:510–5.

[8] Bohm B, Voth M, Geoghegan J, et al. Impact of positron emission tomography on strategy in liver resection for primary and secondary liver tumors. J Cancer Res Clin Oncol 2004;130:266–72.

[9] Vitola JV, Delbeke D, Sandler MP, et al. Positron emission tomography to stage suspected metastatic colorectal carcinoma to the liver. Am J Surg 1996;171: 21–6.

[10] Hustinx R, Paulus P, Jacquet N, et al. Clinical evaluation of whole-body 18F-fluorodeoxyglucose positron emission tomography in the detection of liver metastases. Ann Oncol 1998;9:397–401.

[11] Arulampalam TH, Francis DL, Visvikis D, et al. FDG-PET for the pre-operative evaluation of colorectal liver metastases. Eur J Surg Oncol 2004;30:286–91.

[12] Schiepers C, Penninckx F, De Vadder N, et al. Contribution of PET in the diagnosis of recurrent colorectal cancer: comparison with conventional imaging. Eur J Surg Oncol 1995;21:517–22.

[13] Ogunbiyi OA, Flanagan FL, Dehdashti F, et al. Detection of recurrent and metastatic colorectal cancer: comparison of positron emission tomography and computed tomography. Ann Surg Oncol 1997;4: 613–20.

[14] Fernandez FG, Drebin JA, Linehan DC, et al. Five-year survival after resection of hepatic metastases from colorectal cancer in patients screened by positron emission tomography with F-18 fluorodeoxyglucose (FDG-PET). Ann Surg 2004;240:438–47.

[15] Flanagan FL, Dehdashti F, Ogunbiyi OA, et al. Utility of FDG-PET for investigating unexplained plasma CEA elevation in patients with colorectal cancer. Ann Surg 1998;227:319–23.

[16] Yang M, Martin DR, Karabulut N, et al. Comparison of MR and PET imaging for the evaluation of liver metastases. J Magn Reson Imaging 2003;17:343–9.

[17] Kinkel K, Lu Y, Both M, et al. Detection of hepatic metastases from cancers of the gastrointestinal tract by using noninvasive imaging methods (US, CT, MR imaging, PET): a meta-analysis. Radiology 2002;224: 748–56.

[18] Marom EM, McAdams HP, Erasmus JJ, et al. Staging non-small cell lung cancer with whole-body PET. Radiology 1999;212:803–9.

[19] Topal B, Flamen P, Aerts R, et al. Clinical value of whole-body emission tomography in potentially curable colorectal liver metastases. Eur J Surg Oncol 2001;27:175–9.

[20] Ruers TJ, Langenhoff BS, Neeleman N, et al. Value of positron emission tomography with [F-18]fluorodeoxyglucose in patients with colorectal liver metastases: a prospective study. J Clin Oncol 2002;20:388–95.

[21] Chatziioannou AF. Molecular imaging of small animals with dedicated PET tomographs. Eur J Nucl Med Mol Imaging 2002;29:98–114.

[22] Visvikis D, Ell PJ. Impact of technology on the utilisation of positron emission tomography in lymphoma: current and future perspectives. Eur J Nucl Med Mol Imaging 2003;30(Suppl 1):S106–16.

[23] Zasadny KR, Wahl RL. Enhanced FDG-PET tumor imaging with correlation-coefficient filtered influx-constant images. J Nucl Med 1996;37:371–4.

[24] Rohren EM, Paulson EK, Hagge R, et al. The role of F-18 FDG positron emission tomography in preoperative assessment of the liver in patients being considered for curative resection of hepatic metastases from colorectal cancer. Clin Nucl Med 2002;27:550–5.

[25] Osman MM, Cohade C, Nakamoto Y, et al. Clinically significant inaccurate localization of lesions with PET/CT: frequency in 300 patients. J Nucl Med 2003;44:240–3.

[26] Korin HW, Ehman RL, Riederer SJ, et al. Respiratory kinematics of the upper abdominal organs: a quantitative study. Magn Reson Med 1992;23:172–8.

[27] Weiss PH, Baker JM, Potchen EJ. Assessment of hepatic respiratory excursion. J Nucl Med 1972;13: 758–9.

[28] Nehmeh SA, Erdi YE, Ling CC, et al. Effect of respiratory gating on quantifying PET images of lung cancer. J Nucl Med 2002;43:876–81.

[29] Nakamoto Y, Chin BB, Kraitchman DL, et al. Effects of nonionic intravenous contrast agents at PET/CT imaging: phantom and canine studies. Radiology 2003;227:817–24.

[30] Cohade C, Wahl RL. Applications of positron emission tomography/computed tomography image fusion in clinical positron emission tomography-clinical use, interpretation methods, diagnostic improvements. Semin Nucl Med 2003;33:228–37.

[31] Francis DL, Freeman A, Visvikis D, et al. In vivo imaging of cellular proliferation in colorectal cancer using positron emission tomography. Gut 2003;52: 1602–6.

[32] Francis DL, Visvikis D, Costa DC, et al. Potential impact of [18F]3′-deoxy-3′-fluorothymidine versus [18F]fluoro-2-deoxy-D-glucose in positron emission tomography for colorectal cancer. Eur J Nucl Med Mol Imaging 2003;30:988–94.

[33] Levy AD. Malignant liver tumors. Clin Liver Dis 2002;6:147–64.

[34] el-Serag HB. Epidemiology of hepatocellular carcinoma. Clin Liver Dis 2001;5:87–107.

[35] Ryder SD, British Society of Gastroenterology. Guidelines for the diagnosis and treatment of hepatocellular carcinoma (HCC) in adults. Gut 2003;52(Suppl 3): iii1–8.

[36] Roh MS, Jeong JS, Kim YH, et al. Diagnostic utility of GLUT1 in the differential diagnosis of liver carcinomas. Hepatogastroenterology 2004;51:1315–8.

[37] Iwata Y, Shiomi S, Sasaki N, et al. Clinical usefulness of positron emission tomography with fluorine-18-fluorodeoxyglucose in the diagnosis of liver tumors. Ann Nucl Med 2000;14:121–6.

[38] Schroder O, Trojan J, Zeuzem S, et al. Limited value of fluorine-18-fluorodeoxyglucose PET for the differential diagnosis of focal liver lesions in patients with chronic hepatitis C virus infection. Nuklearmedizin 1998;37:279–85.

[39] Trojan J, Schroeder O, Raedle J, et al. Fluorine-18 FDG positron emission tomography for imaging of hepatocellular carcinoma. Am J Gastroenterol 1999; 94:3314–9.

[40] Okazumi S, Isono K, Enomoto K, et al. Evaluation of liver tumors using fluorine-18-fluorodeoxyglucose PET: characterization of tumor and assessment of effect of treatment. J Nucl Med 1992;33:333–9.

[41] Torizuka T, Tamaki N, Inokuma T, et al. In vivo assessment of glucose metabolism in hepatocellular carcinoma with FDG-PET. J Nucl Med 1995;36: 1811–7.

[42] Shiomi S, Nishiguchi S, Ishizu H, et al. Usefulness of positron emission tomography with fluorine-18-fluorodeoxyglucose for predicting outcome in patients with hepatocellular carcinoma. Am J Gastroenterol 2001;96: 1877–80.

[43] Kong YH, Han CJ, Lee SD, et al. Positron emission tomography with fluorine-18-fluorodeoxyglucose is useful for predicting the prognosis of patients with hepatocellular carcinoma. Korean J Hepatol 2004;10: 279–87.

[44] Lee JD, Yun M, Lee JM, et al. Analysis of gene expression profiles of hepatocellular carcinomas with regard to 18F-fluorodeoxyglucose uptake pattern on positron emission tomography. Eur J Nucl Med Mol Imaging 2004;31:1621–30.

[45] Nakeeb A, Pitt HA, Sohn TA, et al. Cholangiocarcinoma: a spectrum of intrahepatic, perihilar, and distal tumors. Ann Surg 1996;224:463–73.

[46] Pichlmayr R, Weimann A, Klempnauer J, et al. Surgical treatment in proximal bile duct cancer: a single-center experience. Ann Surg 1996;224:628–38.

[47] Zimmerman RL, Fogt F, Burke M, et al. Assessment of Glut-1 expression in cholangiocarcinoma, benign biliary lesions and hepatocellular carcinoma. Oncol Rep 2002;9:689–92.

[48] Kato T, Tsukamoto E, Kuge Y, et al. Clinical role of (18)F-FDG-PET for initial staging of patients with extrahepatic bile duct cancer. Eur J Nucl Med Mol Imaging 2002;29:1047–54.

[49] Kim YJ, Yun M, Lee WJ, et al. Usefulness of 18F-FDG-PET in intrahepatic cholangiocarcinoma. Eur J Nucl Med Mol Imaging 2003;30:1467–72.

[50] Fritscher-Ravens A, Bohuslavizki KH, Broering DC, et al. FDG-PET in the diagnosis of hilar cholangiocarcinoma. Nucl Med Commun 2001;22:1277–85.

[51] Bartolozzi C, Cioni D, Donati F, et al. Focal liver lesions: MR imaging-pathologic correlation. Eur Radiol 2001;11:1374–88.

[52] Misra S, Chaturvedi A, Misra NC, et al. Carcinoma of the gallbladder. Lancet Oncol 2003;4:167–76.

[53] Abi-Rached B, Neugut AI. Diagnostic and management issues in gallbladder carcinoma. Oncology (Huntingt) 1995;9:19–24 [discussion: 24, 27, 30].

[54] Kim YW, Park YK, Yoon TY, et al. Expression of the GLUT1 glucose transporter in gallbladder carcinomas. Hepatogastroenterology 2002;49:907–11.

[55] Koh T, Taniguchi H, Yamaguchi A, et al. Differential diagnosis of gallbladder cancer using positron emission tomography with fluorine-18-labeled fluorodeoxyglucose (FDG-PET). J Surg Oncol 2003;84: 74–81.

[56] Anderson CD, Rice MH, Pinson CW, et al. Fluorodeoxyglucose PET imaging in the evaluation of gallbladder carcinoma and cholangiocarcinoma. J Gastrointest Surg 2004;8:90–7.

[57] Yaeger TE, Brady LW. Basis for current major therapies for cancer. In: Lenhard RE, Osteen RT, Gansler T, editors. The American Cancer Society's clinical oncology. Blackwell Science; 2001. p. 159–229.

[58] Mikhaeel NG, Timothy AR, O'Doherty MJ, et al. 18-FDG-PET as a prognostic indicator in the treatment of aggressive non-Hodgkin's lymphoma-comparison with CT. Leuk Lymphoma 2000;39:543–53.

[59] Friedberg JW, Fischman A, Neuberg D, et al. FDG-PET is superior to gallium scintigraphy in staging and more sensitive in the follow-up of patients with de novo Hodgkin lymphoma: a blinded comparison. Leuk Lymphoma 2004;45:85–92.

[60] Spaepen K, Stroobants S, Dupont P, et al. Early restaging positron emission tomography with (18)F-fluorodeoxyglucose predicts outcome in patients with aggressive non-Hodgkin's lymphoma. Ann Oncol 2002;13:1356–63.

[61] Weber WA, Ott K, Becker K, et al. Prediction of response to preoperative chemotherapy in adenocarcinomas of the esophagogastric junction by metabolic imaging. J Clin Oncol 2001;19:3058–65.

[62] Schelling M, Avril N, Nahrig J, et al. Positron emission tomography using [(18)F]Fluorodeoxyglucose for monitoring primary chemotherapy in breast cancer. J Clin Oncol 2000;18:1689–95.

[63] Smith IC, Welch AE, Hutcheon AW, et al. Positron emission tomography using [(18)F]-fluorodeoxy-D-glucose to predict the pathologic response of breast cancer to primary chemotherapy. J Clin Oncol 2000; 18:1676–88.

[64] Findlay M, Young H, Cunningham D, et al. Non-invasive monitoring of tumor metabolism using

fluorodeoxyglucose and positron emission tomography in colorectal cancer liver metastases: correlation with tumor response to fluorouracil. J Clin Oncol 1996;14: 700–8.

[65] Dimitrakopoulou-Strauss A, Strauss LG, Rudi J. PET-FDG as predictor of therapy response in patients with colorectal carcinoma. Q J Nucl Med 2003;47:8–13.

[66] Goerres GW, Stupp R, Barghouth G, et al. The value of PET, CT and in-line PET/CT in patients with gastrointestinal stromal tumours: long-term outcome of treatment with imatinib mesylate. Eur J Nucl Med Mol Imaging 2005;32:153–62.

[67] McGhana JP, Dodd III GD. Radiofrequency ablation of the liver: current status. AJR Am J Roentgenol 2001;176:3–16.

[68] Livraghi T, Goldberg SN, Lazzaroni S, et al. Hepatocellular carcinoma: radio-frequency ablation of medium and large lesions. Radiology 2001;218: 918–9.

[69] Donckier V, Van Laethem JL, Goldman S, et al. [F-18] fluorodeoxyglucose positron emission tomography as a tool for early recognition of incomplete tumor destruction after radiofrequency ablation for liver metastases. J Surg Oncol 2003;84:215–23.

[70] Torizuka T, Tamaki N, Inokuma T, et al. Value of fluorine-18-FDG-PET to monitor hepatocellular carcinoma after interventional therapy. J Nucl Med 1994; 35:1965–9.

[71] Langenhoff BS, Oyen WJ, Jager GJ, et al. Efficacy of fluorine-18-deoxyglucose positron emission tomography in detecting tumor recurrence after local ablative therapy for liver metastases: a prospective study. J Clin Oncol 2002;20:4453–8.

[72] Morikawa H, Shiomi S, Sasaki N, et al. Hepatocellular carcinoma monitored by F-18 fluorodeoxyglucose positron emission tomography after laparoscopic microwave coagulation therapy. Clin Nucl Med 1999;24: 536–8.

[73] Anderson GS, Brinkmann F, Soulen MC, et al. FDG positron emission tomography in the surveillance of hepatic tumors treated with radiofrequency ablation. Clin Nucl Med 2003;28:192–7.

[74] Wong CY, Salem R, Raman S, et al. Evaluating 90Y-glass microsphere treatment response of unresectable colorectal liver metastases by [18F]FDG-PET: a comparison with CT or MRI. Eur J Nucl Med Mol Imaging 2002;29:815–20.

[75] Wong CY, Salem R, Qing F, et al. Metabolic response after intraarterial 90Y-glass microsphere treatment for colorectal liver metastases: comparison of quantitative and visual analyses by 18F-FDG-PET. J Nucl Med 2004;45:1892–7.

[76] Ishiwata K, Enomoto K, Sasaki T, et al. A feasibility study on L-[1-carbon-11]tyrosine and L-[methyl-carbon-11]methionine to assess liver protein synthesis by PET. J Nucl Med 1996;37:279–85.

ELSEVIER
SAUNDERS

Radiol Clin N Am 43 (2005) 861 – 886

**RADIOLOGIC
CLINICS**
of North America

MR Imaging of the Liver

Diego R. Martin, MD, PhD[a],*, Raman Danrad, MD[a], Shahid M. Hussain, MD[b]

[a]Department of Radiology, Emory University School of Medicine, 1364 Clifton Road NE, Atlanta, GA 30322, USA
[b]Section of Abdominal Imaging, Department of Radiology, Erasmus MC, Dr. Molewaterplein 40,
3015 GD Rotterdam, The Netherlands

MR imaging is establishing a role as a primary diagnostic technique with increasing evidence showing MR imaging to have advantages over CT regarding diagnostic sensitivity and specificity for many pathologies of solid organs, bile and pancreatic ducts, bowel, peritoneum, and retroperitoneum. In addition, there are increasing concerns regarding the risks of radiation and iodinated contrast associated with CT imaging of the abdomen. For example, lifetime risk from a single full-body CT scan for a 45-year-old man has been estimated to be 0.08% [1], whereas the estimated attributable cancer mortality risk from annual CT scans obtained from 45 to 75 years of age is approximately 2%, largely based on estimations derived from Hiroshima atomic bomb victims showing a measurable increased cancer risk related to exposure rates as low as 50 mSv [1]. The incidence of contrast-induced nephropathy associated with iodinated contrast used for CT scanning is difficult to ascertain because reporting is spurious and variable in interpretation. Although the risk of renal insufficiency for the general population is estimated at below 2%, risk factors including pre-existing impaired renal function, diabetes mellitus, and high-contrast administration may significantly elevate the likelihood [2]. Patients with diabetes and mild to moderate renal insufficiency have been estimated to have between a 9% and 40% risk, and this estimated risk has been reported to increase between 50% and 90% in various studies [3,4].

MR imaging techniques and concepts

One of the major challenges of MR imaging in the abdomen has centered on the problem of acquiring data from tissue that has high spatial displacement low-frequency movement, mostly caused by respiratory-dependent movement of the diaphragm. MR imaging of the liver initially relied on standard spin echo T1- and T2-weighted methods, representing sequences that acquire data over a long time window relative to respiratory movement [5–7]. This requires supplemental techniques of respiratory gating, which in turn adds to the total acquisition time. Typical scan times with these techniques can lead to total procedure times in excess of 60 minutes. State-of-the-art MR imaging technique allows shorter acquisition time sequences that can be completed within a breathhold, including T1-weighted fast spoiled gradient echo (SGE) and breathhold half-Fourier transform single shot spin echo methods [6–12]. The single shot spin echo sequences are slice selective, performing all of the preparation and acquisition for an individual slice in approximately 1 second, with the central k-space data acquired over a fraction of that time. Because the image contrast is derived from central k-space, single shot techniques are remarkably motion insensitive, and have breathing-independent characteristics that are useful in noncompliant patients [12]. T1-weighted gradient echo, either two-dimensional or three-dimensional sequences, tend to be motion sensitive because these techniques use interleaved phase lines: the phase lines are collected from each image slice one phase line at a time moving from slice-to-slice. This leads to the observation that even transient motion occurring

---

* Corresponding author.
E-mail address: diego_martin@emoryhealthcare.org
(D.R. Martin).

radiologic.theclinics.com

during only a fraction of the acquisition affects all the slices. T1-weighted techniques with motion-insensitive properties are also available. These use the same basic concept of acquiring two-dimensional data with rapid filling of central k-space by preparing and analyzing one slice at a time, but based on SGE sequences [13–15] using an inversion or saturation prepulse to generate the T1 contrast. These sequences have been referred to as "turbo fast low angle shot" and "fast inversion recovery motion insensitive."

Another development has been the application of three-dimensional gradient echo sequences, modified from MR imaging angiographic techniques, with various vendor-specific names including the first description of this technique called volumetric interpolated breathhold examination [16]. This approach facilitates generation of high-resolution images of the liver, particularly out-of-plane resolution, with ability to generate near isotropic voxel sizes in the order of 2 to 2.5 mm. Such an approach allows better

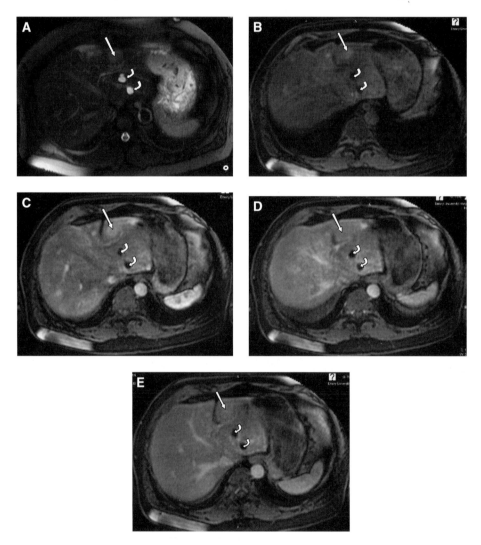

Fig. 1. Hypervascular metastases showing signal characteristics typical for melanoma and a benign cyst demonstrated on the same image. Multiple masses representative of melanoma metastases are shown (*A–E, arrows*). (*A*) Lesions demonstrate elevated signal on T2-weighted single shot spin echo image. (*B*) Lesions demonstrate elevated signal on the T1-weighted gradient echo image, an unusual feature, and characteristic of melanin-containing tumors. Postcontrast arterial (*C*), venous (*D*), and delayed (*E*) enhanced images show transient arterial phase marked enhancement. Two cysts (*curved arrows*) are also seen in the hepatic segment. In contrast to the melanoma metastases, cysts show higher and uniform signal on T2-weighted (*A*) and low signal on T1-weighted images (*B*), with no perceptible enhancement (*C–E*).

evaluation of hepatic vascular anatomy, and generates volumetric data sets that can be used for multiplanar reconstruction. Currently, one of the limitations of high spatial resolution three-dimensional techniques may be related to reduced soft tissue contrast relative to two-dimensional gradient echo sequences acquired with thicker sections. Another useful technique in SGE imaging is the ability to acquire images at two echo-times during a single breathhold, with short echo times set to either capture signal when water and fat environment hydrogen protons are in phase, around 4.2 milliseconds (on a 1.5-T system) resulting in maximal signal, or when these protons are in 180 degree opposed phase, at 2.1 millisecond, resulting in minimal signal. This allows assessment of fat-water composition within soft tissues, which can be useful for characterization of diffuse or focal liver pathologies, such as fatty infiltration or fatty adenomas, respectively.

Another critical element in T1-weighted breathhold imaging is the addition of intravenously administered gadolinium contrast enhancement. Gadolinium chelate is a T1 shortening agent that results in marked elevation of signal on T1-weighted

images, and is used to assess focal liver lesions based on characteristic vascularization (compare lesions shown in Figs. 1–3), which can be distinguished from adjacent normal hepatic parenchyma [16,17]. The liver is unique in having a dual blood supply, receiving 70%– 80% of afferent blood flow from the portal vein, and the remainder from the hepatic artery. Hepatic tumors develop selective portal venous or hepatic arterial blood supply related to characteristics of specific tumors. Tumors that derive blood supply from hepatic arterial branches are best visualized during the hepatic arterial-dominant phase of liver enhancement (Fig. 4). Hypovascular tumors are predominantly supplied by portal venous branches, and demonstrate enhancement-time curves that are different than normal liver, having slower and less intense enhancement, at least partly because of the lack of contribution from the hepatic arterial supply, and partly because of the lower total volume of intravascular volume per gram of tissue (Fig. 5). Over time, measured in units of minutes, the gadolinium concentration may slowly increase in a nonuniform pattern within these tumors because of leakage of contrast into the interstitial spaces. A key to diag-

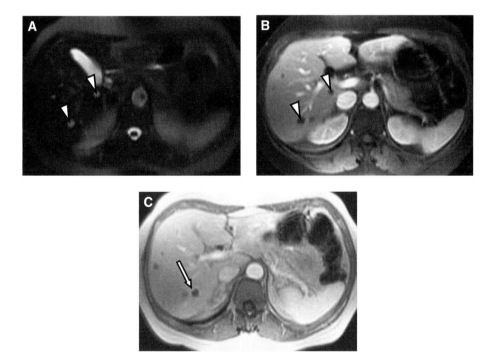

Fig. 2. Hamartoma. (A) T2-weighted single shot spin echo image shows multiple well-defined hyperintense subcentimeter masses predominantly toward the liver periphery (arrowheads). Two-dimensional gradient echo images at 20 (B) and 60 seconds (C) postgadolinium enhancement show subtle thin smooth enhancement circumscribing the periphery of the cysts (arrow). These features are characteristic of biliary hamartoma.

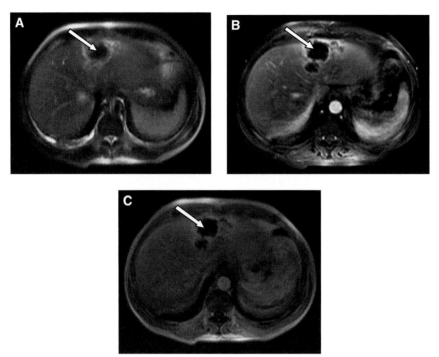

Fig. 3. Hepatic abscess. (*A*) T2-weighted single shot spin echo image shows perilesional high signal consistent with edema. Early (*B*) and late (*C*) gadolinium-enhanced T1-weighted gradient echo images show peripheral and perilesional thick concentric marked enhancement in keeping with reactive inflammatory changes. The lesion center has variable low signal on T2-weighted (*A, arrow*) and no enhancement on postgadolinium T1-weighted (*B* and *C, arrow*) images, in keeping with central necrotic debris.

nostic MR imaging liver examinations is dynamic multiphase postgadolinium SGE imaging, which provides information regarding the time intensity curves of hepatic lesions [8,9,18,19]. Gadolinium chelate is extremely safe, with risk for serious reaction estimated at around 1 per million, and for mild reactions around 2.5%, and is relatively pharmacologically inert with minimal or no well-established adverse renal affects. Although other contrast agents have been developed for imaging of liver lesions, gadolinium remains well established as the most useful. Other products currently available include iron oxide or manganese-based contrast agents [9,20–27]. Superparamagnetic iron oxide particles are taken up by functioning Kupffer cells, concentrating within the intracellular space over time, but not by non-Kupffer cell– containing masses. Iron oxide results in paramagnetic effects that decreases signal in normal liver parenchyma on T2-weighted images, facilitating detection of tumors. Tumors with intermediate to high signal on T2-weighted sequences do not take up contrast and become more conspicuous as the background of normal liver develops progressively lower signal because of uptake of iron oxide. This

contrast agent lacks dynamic enhancement information, reducing the ability to characterize lesions, and can be associated with considerable side effects. Manganese-DPDP, a T1-shortening agent, is taken up by normal hepatocytes through the same transport mechanism used by circulating bile salts, and secreted into the bile duct canaliculi without being metabolized. Adequate liver uptake requires at least 20 minutes delay after intravenous administration and results in elevated signal on T1-weighted SGE images in normal liver and bile ducts, rendering focal liver masses, which lack functional hepatocytes, as relatively lower signal foci. As with iron oxide, manganese-DPDP lacks critical dynamic enhancement characteristics. Furthermore, certain benign and malignant tumors have been shown to take up manganese-DPDP, becoming relatively less conspicuous. Tumors included in this group are benign focal nodular hyperplasia (FNH) and a subset of well-differentiated hepatocellular carcinoma (HCC), and metastatic pancreatic islet cell tumors [9]. It has been shown that the distinct unique beneficial properties of gadolinium and of manganese can be combined during a single patient visit using a protocol based

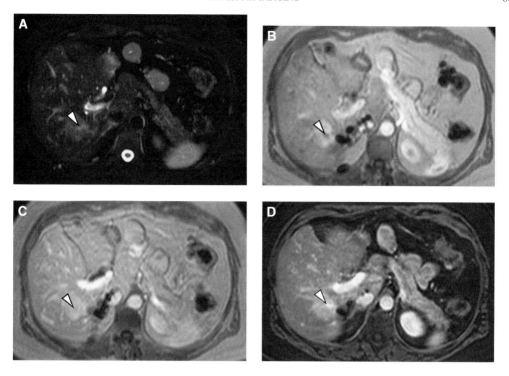

Fig. 4. Focal nodular hyperplasia. (*A*) T2-weighted single shot spin echo image shows a lesion with central irregularly shaped scar having high signal intensity (*arrowhead*). (*B*) The scar (*arrowhead*) does not enhance in early arterial phase, whereas the lesion tissue surrounding the central scar enhances rapidly compared with adjacent liver. (*C*) Enhancement of the lesion and scar is less apparent on the portovenous phase because the adjacent hepatic parenchyma starts to approach peak enhancement. (*D*) Delayed images show intense enhancement of the scar (*arrowhead*) and the remainder of the lesion begins to blend with hepatic parenchyma, but remains slightly hyperintense to adjacent liver in this case. Note no evidence of a peripheral pseudo-capsule on the delayed postgadolinium image (*D*).

on sequential administration of gadolinium during dynamic imaging, followed by manganese [9]. This has similarly been shown for gadolinium and iron oxide particles [24]. Because alternative agents to gadolinium lack in lesion characterization properties, the main reason for their use is to improve lesion detection sensitivity if used in combination with a gadolinium agent. Other contrast agents are being formulated to combine chemically the benefits of the extracellular dynamic enhancing properties of gadolinium with the hepatocyte-specific manganese agent. These include gadolinium-EOB-DTPA and gadolinium-DTPA-BOPTA. Use may be in selected patients where a tumor has nonspecific features even after an optimally performed gadolinium-enhanced study. A specific suggested application is to differentiate an adenoma from FNH. Gadolinium-EOB-DTPA is taken up by hepatocytes and excreted into bile ducts and over a 1 hour period may accumulate within blind-ending poorly draining ducts typical of FNH, but may not accumulate within an adenoma,

fibrolamellar carcinoma, HCC, or hypervascular metastases, facilitating differentiation.

A review of the enhancement characteristics of the benign and malignant lesions reveals that most diagnostically important information can be derived from the hepatic arterial-phase SGE images. Most of the information required for making a specific diagnosis of cyst, hemangioma, hamartoma, hypervascular FNH, or adenoma, or of a hypervascular HCC in cirrhosis versus a hypervascular or hypovascular metastases, is present in the images. The role of T2-weighted imaging is predominantly not lesion detection, but rather lesion characterization, to demonstrate high water content, usually associated with benign cysts, hemangiomas, or bile duct hamartomas. Hypervascular metastases can demonstrate elevated signal on T2-weighted images, however, requiring assessment on hepatic arterial-dominant phase SGE images. It is then the T1-weighted SGE images that can provide most lesion detection sensitivity [9]. The timing delay between initiation of contrast admin-

SGE = spoiled gradient echo

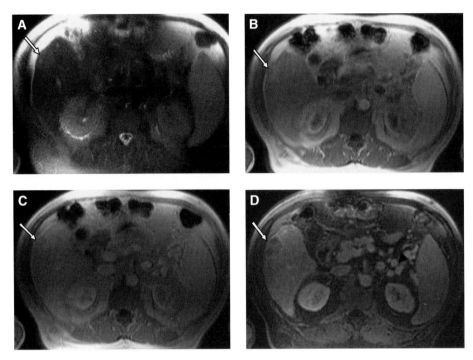

Fig. 5. Cirrhosis and hepatocellular carcinoma. Axial T2-weighted breathhold single shot fast spin echo (*A*), and gadolinium-enhanced SGE T1-weighted arterial (*B*), venous (*C*), and fat-suppressed delayed phase (*D*) images though the liver. A mass (*A–D, arrow*) is shown to have high T2 signal (*A*), and central diffuse enhancement on arterial phase imaging (*B*), with rapid wash-out and peripheral pseudocapsule enhancement developing in the venous (*C*) and equilibrium phase images (*D*). Diffuse fine reticular late enhancement pattern in liver parenchyma is in keeping with cirrhosis (*D*).

istration and initiation of the SGE scan for optimal hepatic arterial-dominant phase SGE images is critical, with a narrow time window of between 18 and 20 seconds noted for most patients. Visually, this can be verified on the resulting images with ideal results showing contrast enhancement of the central portal veins, whereas the hepatic veins remain completely unenhanced. The optimal time for portal venous-dominant phase is less critical, and optimal timing delay is between 45 and 60 seconds, with ideal images showing recent filling of the hepatic veins. The timing delay for delayed-phase images is the least critical, and can be performed anytime between 1.5 and 5 minutes, with no demonstrated benefit routinely to waiting longer, but rather having the undesirable effect of adding unnecessarily to the total scan time for the patient examination. Although the hepatic arterial-dominant phase SGE gadolinium-enhanced images can be diagnostically critical, it is emphasized that one of the great strengths of MR imaging is the availability of multiple sequences, each delineating different components of normal and pathologic tissues providing both anatomic and functional information.

Liver tumor detection and characterization

Table 1 summarizes a pattern recognition approach to liver tumors, applying concepts described previously. Various comparisons of contrast-enhanced CT and MR imaging have been performed showing that MR imaging has significantly better capacity to characterize liver lesions. A study of 89 patients with liver lesions, confirmed by surgical assessment, percutaneous biopsy, or long-term follow-up, showed that more lesions could be detected on MR imaging in 49% of patients, and that in 25% of these cases no lesions were seen on CT, whereas all true-positive lesions identified on CT were also identified on MR imaging [9]. More lesions were characterized in 75% of patients on MR imaging. In 61% of patients, the MR image was assessed as having a greater effect on patient management. There has also been comparison of dual-phase spiral CT [9], performed during hepatic arterial and portal venous phases of contrast enhancement. In 22 patients with either benign or malignant lesions, MR imaging was found to have slightly improved lesion detection sensitivity, but significantly greater lesion

Table 1
MR imaging features of benign and malignant masses

Mass	T1	T2	Enhancement		Other features
			Early (arterial)	Late (venous and delayed)	
Benign					
Cyst	↓↓	↑↑	No enhancement	No enhancement	Well-defined borders
Hamartoma	↓↓	↑↑	Thin rim	Thin rim	<1 cm
Hemangioma	↓↓	↑↑	Peripheral nodules	Nodules coalesce, retain	<1.5-cm lesion may enhance
Focal nodular hyperplasia	↓ to ∅	∅ to ↑	Homogeneous intense, nonenhancing scar	Homogeneous washout, late scar enhancement	Central scar liver is commonly fatty
Adenoma	↓ to ↑	∅ to ↑	Homogeneous intense	Homogeneous washout	Uniform signal loss on out-of-phase T1, larger lesions may bleed
Bacterial abscess	↓↓	↑ to ↑↑	Perilesional enhancement, capsule enhances	Perilesional enhancement fades capsule remains enhanced	Resemble metastases but not progressive lesion enhancement
Regenerative nodules	↓ to ∅	↓ to ∅	Negligible	Negligible	Lesions generally <1.5 cm and homogeneous
Malignant or premalignant neoplasms					
Primary					
Mildly dysplastic nodule	↓ to ↑	—	Minimal	Minimal	Lesions generally <1 cm and homogeneous
Severely dysplastic nodule	↓ to ↑	—	Homogeneous intense	Fade to isointense with liver	Lesions generally <1.5 cm, homogeneous, and no capsule
Small HCC (<3cm)	↓ to ↑	∅ to ↑	Diffuse	Rapid washout	—
Large HCC (>3–5 cm)	↓ to ↑	∅ to ↑	Heterogeneous	Heterogeneous ± foci showing washout	Larger lesions may appear infiltrative, poorly marginated, and demonstrate portal vein invasion
Fibrolamellar carcinoma	↓	↑ to ↑↑	Diffuse radiating bands	Slow washout	Usually >5cm
Cholangiocarcinoma	∅ to ↓	∅ to ↑	Negligible	Progressive heterogeneous	Associated liver atrophy intrahepatic duct dilation
Lymphoma (primary)	↓	↑	Diffuse heterogeneous	Progressive with heterogeneous washout	Resemble HCC, rarely may resemble cholangiocarcinoma
Secondary					
Metastasis	↓	↑	±ring, ±perilesional	Heterogeneous	Mucinous adenoma have moderately to mildly increased T2 and more perilesional enhancement
Hypervascular metastases	↓	↑ to ↑↑	Heterogeneous	Variable washout	Resemble metastases
Lymphoma (secondary)	↓	↑	Ring	Progressive mild enhancement	Resemble metastases

Abbreviations: ↓, mildly decreased signal intensity; ↓↓, moderately decreased signal intensity; ∅, isointense; ↑, mildly increased signal intensity; ↑↑, moderately to mildly increased signal intensity.

characterization. In 41% of patients, it was determined that MR imaging added information considered important to clinical management, and that this was because of information on lesion characterization in all cases. MR imaging consistently characterizes over 95% of detected lesions [9]. This compares favorably with percutaneous biopsy, which typically has a diagnostic yield of only 61%– 67% for liver masses [28–30], regardless of imaging modality used for percutaneous needle guidance. Given that about one quarter of liver lesions detected in patients with a history of malignancy are subsequently determined to be malignant, it may be cost effective to image patients directly using MR imaging in patients requiring tumor staging. In patients with malignancy, the ability to characterize a benign liver lesion can be as important as identifying metastases. For example, small liver cysts are common in adult patients, and are frequently too small for accurate density measurement on CT, but can be resolved and characterized down to even 1-mm size cysts on MR imaging, because of very high signal produced on T2-weighted imaging. Generally, the advantages of MR imaging over CT arise from the greater contrast resolution, and the variety of different soft tissue contrast achieved through implementation of multiple sequences.

Benign lesions

Cysts

Benign lesions of the liver are common in the adult, and cysts represent the most common benign lesion. Pathology typically shows a wall comprised of a single layer of epithelial cells. Etiologies are mostly idiopathic, but cysts may be seen in association with developmental disorders, such as polycystic kidney disease or von Hippel-Lindau disease; infections including echinococcus; or hemorrhage. Cysts appear uniform and high in signal intensity on T2- and low on T1-weighted images, with well-defined margins and no evidence of enhancement on gadolinium-enhanced SGE images (see Fig. 1). Benign cysts may appear slightly complicated with lobulation of borders; septations; and may have elevated signal on SGE T1-weighted images, typically in association with protein or related to prior hemorrhage. As the complexity becomes more prominent, the possibility of other considerations should include bile duct adenoma or adenocarcinoma, and mucinous cystadenocarcinoma of ovarian or other origin, usually bowel or pancreas. These tumors, however, typically show perilesional gadolinium enhancement.

Bile duct hamartomas

These lesions are relatively common, occurring in 3% of the population, and are comprised of irregular branching bile-dilated bile ducts. Bile duct hamartomas are frequently peripheral, multiple, and less than 1 cm in size. These lesions have features identical to cysts on T2- and unenhanced T1-weighted images, with the exception of demonstrating a peripheral thin and uniform rim of gadolinium enhancement (see Fig. 2). Metastases show perilesional enhancement, and hypervascular tumors show central enhancement on arterial phase [19,20].

Abscess

Pyogenic abscess are associated with sepsis, recent bowel surgery, diverticulitis, Crohn's disease, and appendicitis. Fungal microabscesses are more common in immunocompromised patients. Typically, abscess has high central increased signal and intermediate peripheral rim on T2-weighted images. The central portion is low on T1-weighted images and does not enhance on the postcontrast study. The peripheral rim shows persistent late enhancement without centripetal progression of enhancement. There is indistinct perilesional enhancement on the early phase because of hyperemia (see Fig. 3).

Hemangiomas

Hemangiomas are the most common benign liver neoplasm, are multiple in up to 70% of cases, and are found with highest incidence in young adult women. Histology shows a series of vascular lakes and channels, with larger lesions developing areas of thrombosis and fibrosis. Imaging shows moderately elevated signal on single-shot T2-weighted images, typically less intense than demonstrated by simple cysts, and low signal on T1-weighted images. Enhanced images show peripheral interrupted nodules on arterial phase, and this finding is pathognomonic for this pathology. Venous and delayed phases may show progressive enlargement and coalescence of the peripheral nodules with variable degrees of central filling. Smaller lesions generally fill more quickly, and larger lesions are progressively more likely to show slower central filling. Larger giant hemangiomas, usually larger than 5 to 10 cm, typically develop central areas that fail to fill in on delayed enhanced images, and may show central cystic areas that are as bright as simple fluid, such as cerebral spinal fluid, with well-defined margins and no enhancement. Small (less than 1 cm) lesions may fill quickly and be difficult to delineate from other arterial-phase enhancing neoplasms, such as a small HCC or hypervascular metastases. In such cases, the distinguishing features can be found on venous and delayed images, where the other hypervascular neoplasms may typically show washout, while hemangiomas may demonstrate persistent enhancement with signal above that of the adjacent liver parenchyma. Treated metastases have been described as having the possible similarity of enhancing progressively from outside-in; however, the pattern of enhancement does not show peripheral interrupted nodules with coalescence, as is typical of hemangiomas. An optimally timed arterial-phase enhanced image data typically provides the most critical diagnostic information.

Focal nodular hyperplasia

FNH are most commonly seen in young adult women and seem to represent a hamartomatous lesion with a disorganized growth pattern of hepatocytes and ducts that can form an unencapsulated mass with abnormally structured vessels and bile ducts. These lesions may appear isointense to mildly hyperintense on T2-weighted, and isointense to mildly hypointense on T1-weighted images. An important characteristic feature of FNH is the formation of a central fibrovascular core. The fibrovascular core may produce a high signal on T2-weighted images, and represents a unique feature of FNH. On gadolinium-enhanced imaging the fibrovascular core may demonstrate slowly progressive enhancement, with no perceived enhancement on arterial phase, and becoming maximally conspicuous on delayed-phase images (see Fig. 4). This is in contrast to the bulk of the mass surrounding the core that typically enhances uniformly and intensely in the arterial phase, and becomes isointense or slightly hyperintense to surrounding liver on venous and delayed phases. Small lesions (less than 1 to 2 cm) may appear more uniform in enhancement and a fibrovascular core may not be perceived. Other distinguishing features on gadolinium-enhanced imaging from other arterial-phase enhancing tumors include the lack of capsule enhancement, as is observed with adenomas and HCC. Fibrolamellar HCCs are typically large, greater than 10 cm at presentation, but may share features of FNH with the exception that the central scar of fibrolamellar tumors is typically lower than surrounding tumor on T2-weighted images and shows radiating enhancing bands on postgadolinium images. Alternative contrast agents may be helpful in a small fraction of cases that remain ambiguous. Gadolinium-EOB-DTPA may demonstrate an early arterial-phase tumor enhancement and late hepatocellular uptake caused by uptake by hepatocytes within the mass and excretion into poorly draining malformed bile ducts. Manganese or SPIO agents may be taken up by hepatocytes within an FNH and darken the lesion similar to surrounding normal liver. Manganese contrast is no longer available, however, within the United States [19,20].

Adenoma

These are benign neoplasms of epithelial origin with predominant incidence in young women and associated with oral contraceptives, and rarely associated with exogenous anabolic steroids, galactosemia, and glycogen storage disease type Ia. Spontaneous hemorrhage may be related to larger masses, typically greater than 4 to 5 cm in diameter, and can result in presentation with abdominal pain, with a risk of extrahepatic extension and intraperitoneal bleeding. Hepatic adenomas are comprised of sheets of hepatocytes and form a pseudocapsule related to compression of adjacent hepatic parenchyma; however, in contrast to FNH, they do not form bile ducts. T2-weighted images show isointense to slightly hyperintense signal and T1-weighted images show mildly hypointense to mildly hyperintense signal. Opposed-phase SGE T1-weighted images may demonstrate signal drop related to lipid accumulation in approximately half of adenomas. Blood products may result in irregular foci of mixed high or low signal on T1- and T2-weighted images. Gadolinium enhancement is maximal during arterial phase and seen as an arterial-phase blush with rapid fading in the venous and delayed phases to hypointensity or isointensity to adjacent liver, with development of a persistent enhancing rim related to the pseudocapsule. An enhancing scar may be observed in a small subset, but such a scar does not produce high signal on T2-weighted images as seen in FNH. Although most features of adenoma mimic HCC, HCC is usually associated with a background of chronic liver disease changes with evidence of cirrhosis. In patients with HCC risk factors where the liver is normal and tumor markers are negative, however, differentiation may be difficult. The presence of portal venous involvement helps differentiate HCC, and the presence of blood products helps to differentiate adenoma. Hepatic adenomatosis is a rare and separate entity that involves numerous adenomas scattered throughout the liver, and which have malignant potential.

Malignant lesions

Primary hepatocellular carcinoma

HCC are the most common primary liver malignancy and usually occur in the setting of cirrhosis. These tumors are thought to arise from premalignant dysplastic nodules, and dysplastic nodules are thought progressively to dedifferentiate from low- to high-grade histology. Increasing grade of dysplastic nodule is associated with a greater capacity to induce vascular proliferation and preferential blood supply from hepatic arterial branches, and there is potential overlap with higher-grade dysplastic nodule and HCC. HCC occurs as a solitary lesion in 50% of cases, multifocal in 40%, and diffuse in 10%, and is typically greater than 2 cm in diameter, in contrast to dysplastic nodules, which are typically less than 2 cm. Imaging features are variable, but the pattern of elevated signal on T2-weighted images and diminished signal on T1-weighted images increases the likelihood of HCC as compared with dysplastic nodules. In the setting of cirrhosis, however, highly specific imaging features for HCC are reliably found on gadolinium-enhanced SGE images that show irregular marked arterial-phase enhancement with rapidly diminished enhancement on venous and delayed-phase images, and development of a peripheral enhancing rim resulting from a pseudocapsule (see Fig. 5). High-grade dysplastic nodules may show enhancement, but do not develop a pseudocapsule. Diffuse HCC shows irregular T2 and T1, with irregular enhancement that has regions that washout, whereas other regions may persist, and typically can be shown to have portal vein arterial phase–enhancing tumor thrombosis [18].

Hypovascular metastases

Most common malignant hepatic tumors can be further classified as hypovascular or hypervascular based on imaging features. Hypovascular metastases are the most common and usually arise from colon adenocarcinoma. These tumors tend to have mixed arterial and portal venous supply, and usually develop central necrosis presumably because of poor vascular perfusion to the center of enlarging tumors. Hypovascular metastases may have variable T2-weighted images and are usually most conspicuous on pre-gadolinium- and postgadolinium-enhanced SGE T1-weighted images, showing slowly progressive irregular enhancement from outside-in (Fig. 6). Unlike hemangioma, the enhancement on arterial phase is

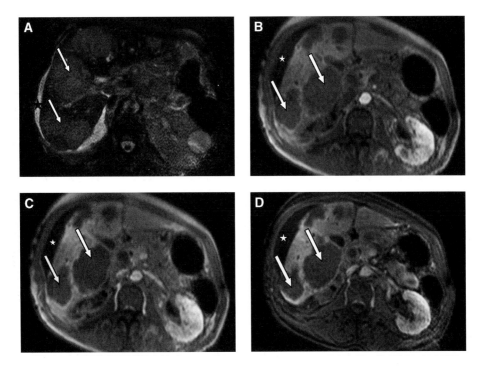

Fig. 6. Hypovascular hepatic metastases from pancreatic adenocarcinoma. (*A*) T2-weighted single shot spin echo image shows hyperintense signal within the central core of multiple metastatic lesions (*arrows*). These metastatic lesions demonstrate course-concentric perilesional enhancement progressively forming on the postgadolinium arterial (*B*), venous (*C*), and delayed (*D*) images. Central tumor does not enhance, and is consistent with central ischemia and necrosis. It is the relative low enhancement of the central region of the masses that designates the characteristics of a hypovascular tumor. The higher signal on T2-weighted imaging is presumably a result of necrotic tissue and relative higher water content. Note perihepatic ascitis, hyperintense on T2-weighted image (*A, black star*) and hypointense on T1-weighted images (*B–D, white star*).

less and does not show peripheral interrupted nodular enhancement. Arterial-phase perilesional enhancement may be observed, and is typically seen with colon, pancreatic, or stomach adenocarcinoma metastases [19,20].

Hypervascular metastases

Hypervascular metastases most commonly are related to carcinoid, or kidney origin, but include pancreatic islet cell tumors and melanoma. T2-weighted images show variable signal, usually moderately elevated, and low signal on T1-weighted images. Melanoma is an exception, where melanin accumulation, having T1 shortening properties, may result in elevated signal on T1-weighted images (see Fig. 1). Characteristic gadolinium enhancement shows that the lesions demonstrate maximal conspicuity on arterial-phase images (Fig. 7) [20].

Malignant mass posttherapy

Cross-sectional imaging has largely relied on anatomic depiction of disease, including tumors. There is a large subset of patients with malignancy being treated by nonsurgical approaches, including chemotherapy and radiation, where the ability to follow tumor response is valuable. Current methods have mostly relied on anatomic depiction of tumor, and measurement of tumor size to evaluate tumor response. This is believed to require a relatively long follow-up period in most applications, and other measures of tumor response sensitive to cellular and vascular reactions may be more useful. A multitude of approaches are being evaluated using MR imaging. One simple test that may be helpful is the evaluation of perfusion by gadolinium enhancement pattern within a treated malignant mass. Demonstration of decreased vascularity posttherapy has been associated with tumor response (Fig. 8) [31].

MR imaging of diffuse liver diseases

It is the objective of all cross-sectional imaging techniques to have the ability to evaluate the anatomic configuration of normal and abnormal tissues. In addition, it has become increasingly evident that

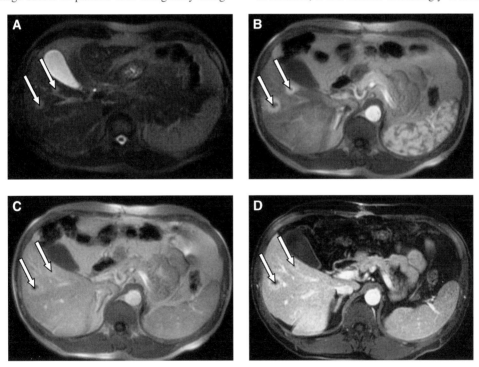

Fig. 7. Hypervascular metastasis from renal cell carcinoma. (*A*) T2-weighted single shot spin echo image shows two hyperintense masses (*arrows*). (*B*) Arterial-phase gadolinium-enhanced T1-weighted gradient echo image shows immediate enhancement of the metastases, which persists, although with slight decrease in conspicuity in the venous (*C*) and delayed (*D*) phases as the hepatic parenchyma reaches peak enhancement. This is consistent with predominant hepatic arterial supply and relatively well-vascularized tissue within the metastatic foci. Elevated tumor signal on T2-weighted image may result from the high vascular content.

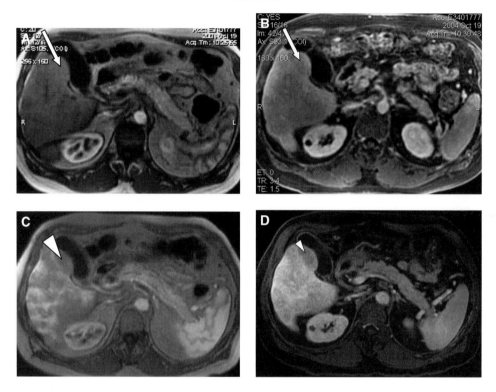

Fig. 8. HCC immediately before and 3 weeks postchemoembolization therapy with early tumor response shown on gadolinium-enhanced images. HCC, demonstrated as a subcapsular mass located in segment 5 and pushing into the gallbladder fossa, enhances as a diffuse blush on arterial phase (*A, arrow*), with rapid washout and formation of pseudocapsule enhancement on delayed (*B, arrow*) gadolinium-enhanced images. Postchemotherapy arterial (*C, arrowhead*) and delayed-phase (*D, arrowhead*) enhanced images show change with no enhancement centrally on the arterial phase (*C*), and a more coarse peripheral lesion enhancement developing on delayed phase (*D*). Before chemoembolization, the liver enhances with a cirrhotic morphology, showing a fine reticular pattern of delayed-phase enhancement, a finding associated with fibrotic changes (*B*). After emboliza-tion therapy, there is marked change in the liver enhancement, developing irregular geographic small foci of bright early enhancement within the liver (*C* versus *A*), with peripheral predominance, becoming diffusely irregular with coarse bands of elevated enhancement on the delayed phase (*D* versus *B*). It is theorized that these features may result from perfusion changes in response to small vessel embolization in a nonuniform distribution, with possible superimposition of reactive inflammatory changes.

MR imaging can demonstrate normal and pathologic processes that represent tissue cellular and intracel-lular architecture, and intracellular processes. Using intravenously injected contrast agent can further pro-vide information regarding the vessels perfusing nor-mal and abnormal tissues, in regards to the origin of the vessels, the number and size of vessels, and the integrity of the vessel walls. Although CT and ul-trasound have some of the abilities found in MR im-aging, the examples discussed in this article show applications of MR imaging of the liver that are uniquely suited to MR imaging, where the combina-tion of different sequences that comprise a routine MR imaging examination are capable of elucidating important and common disease processes and that MR imaging is an evolving anatomic and molecu-lar imaging tool with the capacity to allow realization of the aim to have techniques that represent non-invasive pathology assessment.

The routine MR imaging examination of the liver should use a combination of single shot T2-weighted and breathhold T1-weighted images, and include gadolinium enhancement with acquisition of multiple phases. MR imaging provides superior character-ization of liver masses than CT, and multiphase gadolinium enhancement including a properly timed arterial phase is critical. The T1-weighted precontrast images must include in-phase and out-of-phase acquisitions to assess hepatic lipid or iron content, and dynamically enhanced postgadolinium images. Timing of the arterial-phase images is also critical for demonstration of acute hepatitis. The timing of the venous and equilibrium phase image is less critical, and important for grading more severe acute hepatitis, demonstration of fibrosis, and for delineating vascular abnormalities. In cirrhosis, dynamic postgadolinium images are critical for detection and characterization of regenerative or dysplastic nodules and HCC. The same sequences useful for liver evaluation provide a comprehensive evaluation of all the soft tissues of the abdomen, and allow depiction of most of the important diseases, facilitating use of a universal protocol for abdominal imaging.

The following sections discuss MR imaging sequences for examination of the liver used for the evaluation of diffuse liver diseases, including processes leading to abnormal lipid metabolization; iron deposition disease; and perfusion abnormalities related to inflammation, fibrosis, vascular occlusion, or infarction and hemorrhage.

Fatty liver

Lipid accumulation in hepatocytes can occur as a result of impaired liver function secondary to a variety of etiologies [32]. In the United States, fatty liver can be detected in over 20% of the population, and the most common association with fatty liver is obesity. There has been further association of fatty liver with development of hepatitis, resulting from nonalcoholic acute steatohepatitis, and potential progression to cirrhosis. In the setting of liver transplantation, a living related donor liver assessment must include evaluation for the presence of fatty infiltration, which is considered a contraindication to transplantation when severe and can lead to failure of the transplant.

Abnormal lipid accumulation in liver can be detected on MR imaging [7–11], and can be evaluated on the basis of comparing liver signal on SGE images acquired in-phase and out-of-phase. Hydrogen protons in a voxel containing 100% fat process 220 to 230 Hz slower than a voxel comprised of 100% water at 1.5 T. That means every 4.4 milliseconds the fat protons migrate 360 degrees, and regain in-phase orientation relative to water protons, whereas at 2.2 mil-

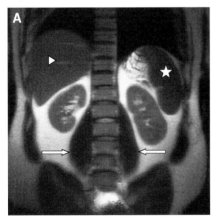
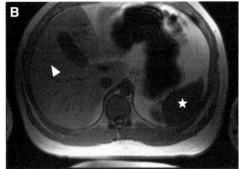
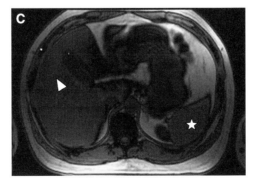

Fig. 9. Hepatic steatosis. On T2-weighted single shot spin echo images liver normally has signal intensity midway between muscle and normal spleen. In this patient, coronal T2-weighted single shot fast spin echo image (*A*) shows liver signal (*arrowhead*) is greater than psoas muscle (*arrows*), and abnormally greater than spleen (*star*). Liver signal diffusely diminishes in signal intensity comparing transverse in-phase (*B*) with out-of-phase (*C*) images of liver, in relation to spleen.

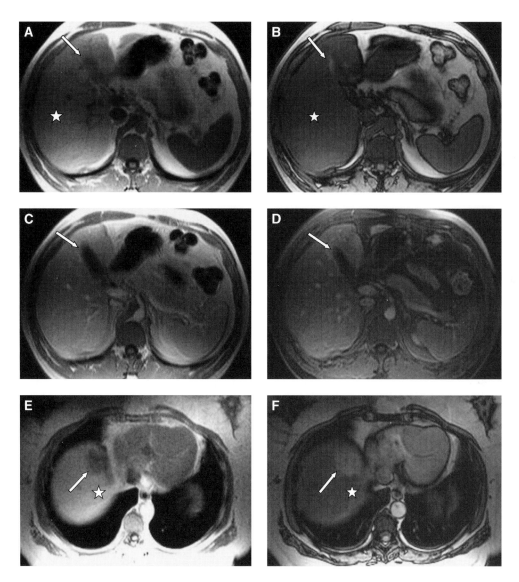

Fig. 10. Steatotic liver with focal sparing in two different patients. (*A – D*) A patient with physiologic focal fatty sparing adjacent to the gallbladder fossa. Axial breathhold in-phase SGE image (*A*) shows normal liver (*star*) and gallbladder fossa (*arrow*). On out-of-phase SGE imaging (*B*), there is marked reduction of liver signal indicating fatty infiltration. The region surrounding the gallbladder fossa shows no signal drop (*arrow*) appearing higher in signal than adjacent fatty liver, representing focal fatty sparing. (*C*) Postgadolinium in-phase SGE (TR/TE of 180/4.2 millisecond) shows normal signal enhancement around the gallbladder fossa (*arrow*). (*D*) On three-dimensional volumetric interpolated breathhold examination SGE postgadolinium imaging (TR/TE of 3.7/1.7 millisecond) shows apparent increased enhancement surrounding the gallbladder fossa (*arrow*). This perception results from postgadolinium imaging using a sequence with out-of-phase TE, and shows the possible confounding effect in the setting of variable fatty infiltration. (*E – G*) Another cause for focal fatty sparing is shown in a different patient. Diffuse fatty infiltration is demonstrated on comparison of in-phase (*E*) with out-of-phase (*F*) axial SGE images. There is a mass (*arrow*) that has low T1-weighted signal relative to normal liver on in-phase imaging (*E*), but demonstrates high signal relative to adjacent liver parenchyma on out-of-phase imaging (*F*). Hepatocytes accumulate intracellular lipid, whereas a tumor lacking hepatocytes does not accumulate lipid, resulting in focal fatty sparing within the mass. In this case, the mass demonstrates peripheral interrupted nodular enhancement on postgadolinium in-phase imaging (*G*) typical of a benign hemangioma. Star, normal liver.

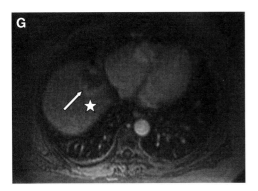

Fig. 10 (*continued*).

liseconds, or at half this time, the fat and water protons are 180 degrees out-of-phase. Current generation MR imaging systems have incorporated dual-echo breathhold SGE sequences that can acquire two sets of k-space filled to obtain two sets of images, one set in-phase, the other out-of-phase, with spatially matched slices. Liver containing lipid results in image voxels with a physical mixture of water and lipid, which when imaged out-of-phase results in phase cancellation and diminished signal (Fig. 9). Spleen is an organ that does not accumulate fat, and can be used as a control against which liver signal can be assessed as a ratio to test for relative diminishment in liver signal on out-of-phase images. Spleen signal can change as a result of iron deposition, and use of kidney or skeletal muscle within the image may be more reliable for assessment of relative liver signal changes between in-phase and out-of-phase images. Fat accumulation in liver can be diffuse (see Fig. 8), diffuse with focal sparing (Fig. 10), or focal. Typical regions affected by focal fatty accumulation occur around the falciform ligament, gallbladder fossa (Fig. 10), and around the inferior vena cava. One possible explanation is that these are areas of liver prone to irritation or stimulation, resulting in changes in local changes in carbohydrate-lipid metabolism. Contrast-enhanced CT and standard ultrasound are relatively nonspecific and less sensitive for assessment of fatty liver, and can confuse irregularly accumulated lipid with a mass [6,10,14–22]. Fatty liver can lead to reduced CT density, and diminish contrast between a low-density mass [31,33,34] and adjacent liver, making the mass less conspicuous [31,32,35].

Iron deposition disease

Iron can accumulate within the liver through two basic mechanisms: accumulation within hepatocytes through normal metabolic chelation mechanisms; or through uptake within the phagocytic Kupffer cells, representing part of the reticuloendothelial system [36]. Serum iron and transferrin saturation are poorly correlated with the degree of iron overload. Although serum ferritin can be used to estimate body iron stores, a variety of etiologies can lead to elevation of serum levels, independent of total body iron.

In primary hemochromatosis, the defect seems to be caused by inappropriately regulated small bowel increased uptake of dietary iron, resulting in excess total body iron accumulation [36]. Hepatocytes chelate the iron that accumulates within the cytosol. Pancreas also has chelation mechanisms within acinar cells, and can accumulate excess intracellular iron [28]. To some degree, however, iron accumulation can occur in most tissues, typically as a late feature occurring after hepatic stores have reached high levels [26]. Important examples include the pituitary and heart, where this can result in impaired pituitary function and fatal cardiac arrhythmias and congestive heart failure. Patients presenting with a first-time diagnosis of primary hemochromatosis with the combined findings of elevated liver and cardiac iron deposition, and congestive heart failure, have a poor prognosis with a 6-month life-expectancy [37]. There has been rapid recent development of understanding of the genetic basis of this disease, and that there is a defective genetic hemochromatosis gene. The defective genetic hemochromatosis gene seems to represent the most common inherited genetically communicated disease among people of European descent, and has approximately a 1-in-40 occurrence among Americans, with a 1-in-400 incidence of homozygosity [32]. The phenotypic expression of this disease is more complicated, however, and seems to follow a polygenetic penetrance pattern. There is now a clinically available genetic test available that can be used for screening purposes, which is relatively inexpensive.

In secondary hemochromatosis, iron overload can occur secondary to excess red cell turnover from exogenously derived red cells as a result of blood transfusion therapy, as seen in patients with underlying red cell or bone marrow abnormalities, such as thalassemia, mastocytosis, or myelofibrosis. Alternatively, endogenously derived excess iron from red cell turnover can result from polycythemia rubra vera or from myoglobin in rhabdomyolysis, or from siderosis related to alcoholic liver disease. In secondary hemochromatosis, the mechanism of iron accumulation is different than in primary hemochromatosis, resulting from increased uptake of iron derived from hemoglobin arising from dying or abnormal red cells taken up by the reticuloendothelial system, leading to iron accumulation in Kupffer cells within liver sinusoids. Similarly, the splenic reticuloendothelial system phagocytoses abnormal red cells and actively accumulates iron from hemoglobin. In contrast to primary hemochromatosis, the pancreas does not typically accumulate iron. Clinical significance of hemochromatosis includes the observation that many patients develop cirrhosis and approximately 25% of patients develop HCC. These processes also may be evaluated by MR imaging of the liver.

Liver biopsy has been used for biochemical determination of liver iron overload and has been used as the basis for therapy management in patients treated by periodic phlebotomy and iron chelation therapy, but this method has bleeding risks associated with the invasive procedure, and is susceptible to sampling error in patients with heterogeneous iron deposition in the liver. The sensitivity of CT is insufficient, with a minimum threshold for liver iron detection greater than five times above the normal liver iron load, particularly in cases with fatty liver.

MR imaging is sensitive to iron concentration in the liver caused by paramagnetic properties of iron, resulting T2 or T2-star effects that diminish the signal intensity on both single shot breathhold T2 images (Fig. 11) and on breathhold T1-weighted multiecho SGE images [34,37–43]. Quantitative assessment of liver iron concentration based on MR imaging has been demonstrated using both SGE and spin echo

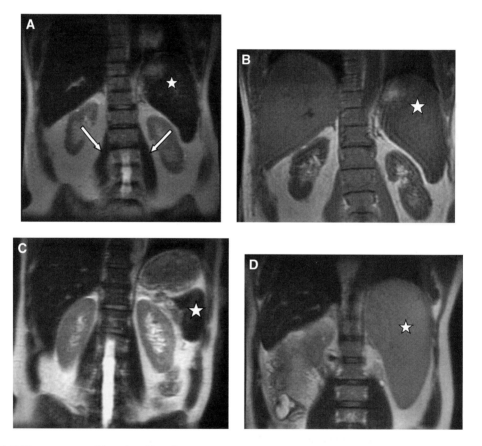

Fig. 11. Different patterns of iron deposition disease in three different patients: bone marrow transplantation blood transfusions and hemosiderosis (A and B); myelofibrosis (C); and hemochromatosis with cirrhosis (D). Coronal imaging facilitates comparison of liver psoas muscle (A, arrows) and spleen (A–D, star). (A and B) The first case, coronal T2-weighted breathhold single shot spin echo imaging shows marked diminished signal in liver and spleen (star) compared with psoas muscle (arrow), whereas abnormal signal is less apparent on T1-weighted breathhold SGE (TR/TE of 180/4.2 millisecond) imaging. In myelofibrosis, both liver and spleen are dark secondary to repeated blood transfusions leading to siderosis with deposition of iron in both liver Kupffer cells and in the reticuloendothelial system of the spleen. In addition, bone marrow expansion and fibrosis replace normal fat and lead to marked diminished signal in the spine (C). The third case (D) shows a dark liver, with splenomegaly secondary to cirrhosis and portal venous hypertension. Hemochromatosis in this case preferentially affects the liver, whereas the spleen (star) retains normal signal.

sequences, relying on measurements of T2-star and T2 decay. Coronal breathhold T2-weighted single shot fast spin echo images, which should be obtained as part of a routine abdominal MR imaging examination, are very useful for rapid visual evaluation, providing slices that include liver, psoas muscle, and spleen within the same image (see Fig. 10). Normally, liver signal intensity is near the midpoint between the lower signal intensity of muscle, and the higher signal intensity of spleen. In iron overload disease, the liver signal intensity becomes as low as or lower than skeletal muscle. In secondary iron overload, spleen similarly becomes dark. In cases where there is bone marrow abnormality, such as in myelofibrosis (see Fig. 11), normal high signal marrow fat becomes replaced with low signal cellular marrow hypertrophy and sclerosis. Chronic iron overload can lead to cirrhosis and increase risk for HCC, complications that can be assessed on MR imaging. For more sensitive and potentially quantitative noninvasive measurement of liver iron, T2-star and T2 decay rate measurements can be performed [44,45]. T2-star decay is a measure of how quickly protons loose phase coherence without use of refocusing pulses, and T2 decay is a measure of proton-dephasing rates after application of refocusing pulses, measuring only dephasing affects that are not correctable. Generally, the T2-star decay rate is more sensitive to lower levels of intracellular iron accumulation. Intracellular iron accumulation can cause localized magnetic field distortion that leads to susceptibility affects, which results in more rapid loss of phase-dependent signal. One method used to detect this affect is based on multiecho gradient echo imaging to measure T2-star decay, whereas a spin echo single shot or echo-planar technique with increasing echo times may be used for T2 decay measurements. When performing imaging dedicated to iron measurement, a series of gradient echo images are acquired with increasing increments of echo-time (TE). As the TE lengthens, the proton dephasing leads to progressive increased loss of signal intensity, and this process has been shown to be proportionately increased in relation to intracellular liver iron concentration. When performing a dedicated T2-star analysis of liver iron, the TEs may be selected to correspond to in-phase echoes, to avoid potential out-of-phase affects from fat, a potential spurious affect in the setting of fatty liver infiltration. At minimum, however, routine imaging of the abdomen and liver should include a dual-echo SGE acquisition (see Fig. 11) that can be used in conjunction with the coronal single shot T2. The longer second echo image (TE of 4.4 milliseconds) should show darkening of the liver, compared with the shorter echo image (TE of 2.2 milliseconds) in the setting of elevated liver iron concentration (see Fig. 11). The sensitivity to liver iron may be increased on SGE imaging by increasing the echo time to include, for example, echoes at 8.8 and 13.2 milliseconds. If only routine shortest possible dual echo out-of-phase (TE of 2.2 milliseconds) and in-phase (TE of 4.4 milliseconds) imaging is used, then the relative sensitivity of the single shot spin echo technique is more sensitive. With this approach, demonstration of low liver signal on single shot spin echo alone indicates a relatively lower liver iron concentration, and demonstration of low liver signal on both single shot spin echo and on the longer echo dual echo SGE indicates relatively higher liver iron burden. Others have shown that liver iron concentration may be calculated and that noninvasive tissue iron concentration may be feasible. This represents the only noninvasive technique available for liver iron quantitation, and could be used, for example, for following hemochromatosis patients on therapy, minimizing the need for liver biopsy. Although it is tempting to suggest the use of MR imaging for genetic hemochromatosis screening, it has been noted that the recent development of a genetic marker test is accurate and relatively inexpensive. Regardless, the ability to determine tissue iron concentration quantitatively by MR imaging is a clinically valuable test, and there are attempts to develop useful methodology for routine clinical imaging [44,45].

Acute hepatitis

Inflammatory liver disease can result from a large number of etiologies, including idiopathic, drug-induced, viral, alcoholic, and gallstone bile duct obstruction [46–48]. It has been noted that MR imaging may be sensitive to acute hepatitis [49]. On MR imaging, the most sensitive images are the post-gadolinium breathhold SGE images acquired during arterial phase (Fig. 12) [46,49]. In a recent report [49] this abnormal enhancement becomes more marked and can persist into the venous and delayed phases as the severity of disease increases, and can resolve in cases when the hepatitis resolves. Furthermore, the arterial-phase timing critically determines sensitivity to mild acute hepatitis. By performing SGE imaging every 5 seconds after administration of gadolinium in a patient with mild acute hepatitis, the authors found that irregular liver enhancement was detectable only during the time when the portal veins were filling with contrast, and the hepatic veins were still unenhanced. In mild hepatitis cases, images acquired before portal venous filling were too early, and

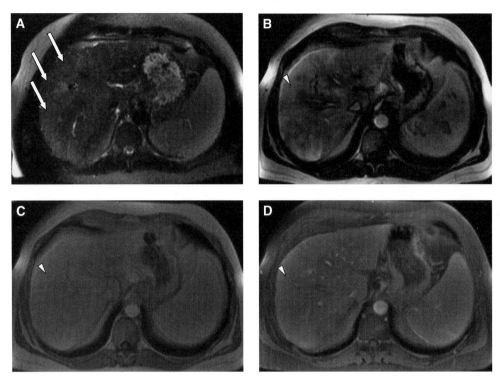

Fig. 12. Viral hepatitis. (*A*) T2-weighted single shot spin echo image shows patchy hyperintensity (*arrows*) in the peripheral right lobe. (*B*) Postcontrast gradient echo image shows patchy peripheral irregular enhancement (*arrowhead*) on the 20-second arterial phase image caused by preferential perfusion from hepatic artery. (*C*) A 60-minute postcontrast image shows patchy enhancement (*arrowhead*) has blended with the rest of the normally enhancing liver parenchyma. (*D*) A 3-minute postcontrast image shows uniform normal enhancement (*arrowhead*).

images acquired when the hepatic veins were filled were too late. For most patients, optimal timing falls between 18 and 22 seconds after initiation of the gadolinium injection into an antecubital vein, administered at 2 mL per second, followed by a 20 mL saline wash-in bolus. The parameters for the breath-hold SGE acquisition must also be taken into account, with the previously mentioned timing based on a gradient echo sequence using linear ordering of k-space, which fills central k-space in the middle of the acquisition time, with a total acquisition time of 18 seconds. If, for example, the acquisition scan time is decreased by 4 seconds to 14 seconds, then the delay time between the start of the injection and the start of the acquisition should be increased by 2 seconds (eg, from 20 to 22 seconds). This ensures that the center lines of k-space are filled at the peak of the hepatic arterial tissue perfusion phase. Conversely, if the acquisition time is increased by 4 seconds to 22 seconds scan time, the delay should be decreased by 2 seconds to 18 seconds. The authors have found that there is an approximately 3- to 4-second window before and after the optimal peak, beyond which an

abnormality seen only during the arterial phase of enhancement may become inconspicuous.

It should be emphasized that no other imaging technique has been shown sensitive for detection of acute hepatitis, and that the authors have previously relied on serum liver enzyme levels, in combination with percutaneous liver biopsy. MR imaging could be used as a diagnostic aid in patients with equivocal liver enzyme elevation and nonspecific symptoms, and in patients presenting with fatty infiltration. Findings suggestive of acute hepatitis, seen as irregular arterial-phase gadolinium enhancement, in the setting of fatty liver, seen as signal drop on out-of-phase gradient echo images, are consistent with steatohepatitis and raise the possible diagnosis of nonalcoholic steatohepatitis or nonalcoholic acute steatohepatitis. Nonalcoholic acute steatohepatitis is a relatively recently recognized disease entity thought to represent a hepatitis that is directly related to excess intracellular fat accumulation within hepatocytes. This disease has strong association with obesity and has a risk of progression to chronic hepatitis and cirrhosis. Given that obesity is an epidemic in the United States, the health concern regarding nonalcoholic acute steatohepatitis is significant. MR imaging has greater sensitivity and specificity for detection of fatty liver, and is the only imaging test sensitive for milder cases of hepatitis as compared with CT or ultrasound.

Multiple causes of transient hepatic perfusion abnormalities have been described [6,11,13]; however, in cases presenting clinically with right upper quadrant pain and abnormal liver arterial-phase perfusion, as described in this study, acute hepatitis should be the major diagnostic consideration. It may be argued that patients with right upper quadrant abdominal symptoms are preferentially examined by MR imaging over CT. MR imaging has potential relative strengths in regards to contrast sensitivity, and can provide excellent temporal resolution because of the small contrast volume used, in combination with the acquisition of contrast data for the entire liver over approximately a 4- to 5-second period, usually in the center of a

two-dimensional T1-weighted gradient echo sequence using interleaved phase acquisition [12]. The safety profile of gadolinium agents and nonionizing radiation imaging for a multiphase examination are also attractive characteristics of MR imaging. A three-dimensional gradient echo T1-weighted sequence may used here for the arterial or venous phase of the examination, with the same potential advantages of temporal resolution. It may be that the relative contrast sensitivity may not be as high as for the three-dimensional gradient echo technique, however, particularly if only thinner slicing reconstructions are used for the three-dimensional technique.

The reasons for heterogeneous liver enhancement in acute hepatitis have not been fully determined. Hypothetically, it may be that the areas of relative arterial-phase hyperenhancement represent regions of abnormality. In this case, periportal inflammation may compress differentially the lower pressure portal vein intrahepatic branches leading to preferential

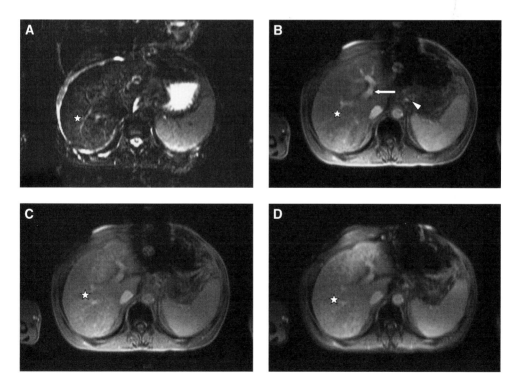

Fig. 13. Active cirrhosis. Axial breathhold T2-weighted single shot fast spin echo (*A*), and breathhold T1-weighted SGE arterial phase (*B*), venous phase (*C*), and fat-suppressed delayed-phase (*D*) images through the liver. T2-weighted image (*A, star*) shows irregular increased signal with areas of linear and reticular pattern toward the periphery (*B, star*), indicating areas of edema, which corresponds to coarse linear and fine reticular patterns of enhancement that progressively increases in delayed venous and equilibrium phase images (*B–D, star*), consistent with areas of late-enhancing fibrosis. Numerous tiny parenchymal liver nodules measuring 3–4 mm mildly enhance in the venous phase (*B, star*) and persist into the equilibrium phase (*D, star*), consistent with small regenerative nodules that derive predominant blood supply from the portal vein. The portal veins are prominent (*B, arrow*), and paraesophageal varices are present (*B, arrowhead*) in this patient with portal hypertension.

segmental hepatic arterial perfusion. Alternatively, the inflammation may lead to altered vascular regulatory affects, with vasodilation and increased hepatic arterial flow to the involved regions. Pathologic correlation is challenging given that histopathologic correlation lacks the ability to determine pathophysiologic in vivo processes involved in hemodynamics, an advantage inherent to contrast-enhanced imaging.

Chronic hepatitis and cirrhosis

A major complication of chronic hepatitis is cirrhosis [46]. In Western nations, the most common etiology has been alcohol-induced hepatitis, but currently viral hepatitis has become the most common cause, and globally viral hepatitis is the most common association with chronic hepatitis, cirrhosis, and HCC.

MR imaging features of fibrosis associated with cirrhosis is progressive enhancement on delayed images [46] (Fig. 13), resulting from leakage of gadolinium contrast agent from the intravascular into the interstitial space within the fibrotic regions. The typical patterns of cirrhosis include fine reticular and coarse linear, with these fibrotic bands outlining foci of regenerative nodules (see Fig. 13). If active hepatitis is present, the fibrotic tissue bands may have edema, and appear high in signal on T2-weighted images [46], and the liver tissue may develop irregular patchy areas of enhancement seen mostly on the arterial phase images.

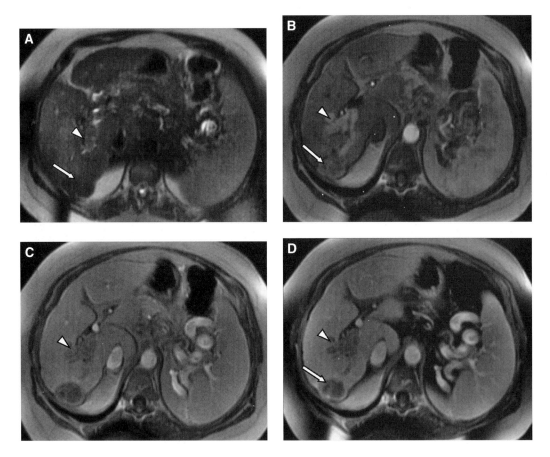

Fig. 14. HCC with portal vein invasion. (*A*) Hypointense mass (*arrow*) is seen in the hepatic segment 6 on T2-weighted single shot spin echo image. Note nodular appearance of the right portal vein branches (*arrowhead*). A subset of HCC can be hypointense on T2-weighted images, although most are typically hyperintense on T2-weighted images. (*B*) There is heterogeneous enhancement of the mass on 20-second gadolinium-enhanced image (*arrow*). Serpiginous enhancement of the right portal vein branches (*arrowhead*) on the arterial phase is characteristic of tumor vascular invasion in keeping with characteristic arterial supply of the tumor. (*C*) There is washout of the tumor and vascular invasion (*arrowhead*) in the portovenous phase. (*D*) Development of ring enhancement (*arrow*) is pathognomic of HCC. The absence of contrast in the branches of the right portal vein (*arrowhead*) while the hepatic veins are opacified demonstrates occlusive thrombus.

Regenerative nodules occur in the setting of cirrhosis [50,51], and represent relatively more normal hepatic parenchyma that derives the major blood supply from the portal venous system. These nodules maximally enhance during portal venous phase postgadolinium SGE images, and are usually less than 1 cm in diameter [42]. These nodules can accumulate iron, and appear low in signal on both SGE T1-, and single shot fast spin echo T2-weighted images, with little enhancement appreciated on postgadolinium SGE images [46].

Dysplastic nodules are premalignant, and are believed to have the potential to transform into progressively higher grades of dysplasia, and finally into HCC. Dysplastic nodules are typically larger than regenerative nodules, and can be seen to grow over a period of weeks or months. These lesions can show overlap with HCC, and may show mildly

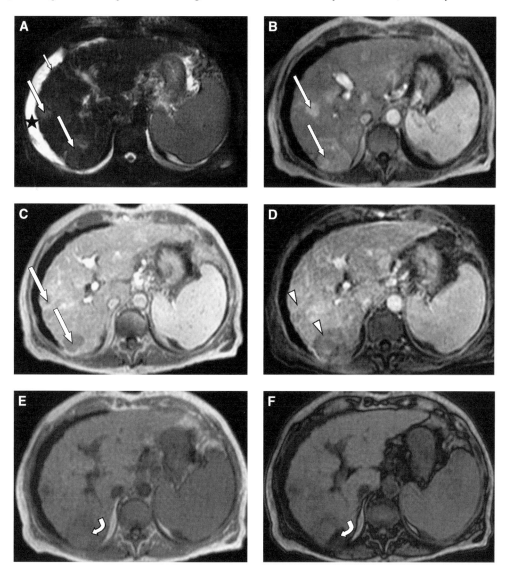

Fig. 15. Atypical fat containing HCC. (*A*) T2-weighted single shot spin echo image shows two hyperintense masses (*large arrows*) noted in right hepatic lobe. There is ascites (*star*) and liver is cirrhotic with a nodular surface (*small arrow*). On comparison with precontrast study (*B*), *C* and *D* show diffuse enhancement of masses at 20- and 60-second postgadolinium enhanced imaging, respectively. (*D*) There is wash out and ring enhancement (*arrowheads*) on 3-minute postcontrast three-dimensional THRIVE images, thought to represent enhancing pseudocapsule. (*E* and *F*) The opposed phase image shows dropout of signal (*arrow*) in comparison with the in-phase image, identifying fat content in HCC.

elevated T1-weighted signal and low T2-weighted signal. Features that help distinguish HCC (Figs. 14 and 15) include elevated T2-weighted signal, transient marked arterial-phase postgadolinium enhancement, capsular peripheral rim enhancement on venous- and equilibrium-phase images, and size greater than 2 to 3 cm. It may be that higher-grade dysplastic nodules overlap more with the HCC features; however, this distinction may be of small clinical significance because the higher-grade dysplasia has the potential of transforming to HCC rapidly. HCC frequently invade vessels and a small subset may contain fat (see Figs. 14 and 15).

Portal hypertension may result from obstruction at presinusoidal, sinusoidal, postsinusoidal, or a combination of these sites corresponding to abnormalities of portal venous, hepatic fibrosis, hepatic venous, or mixed diseases [52]. MR images optimal for visualizing changes related to portal hypertension are obtained on equilibrium-phase SGE images with fat

suppression. In early or mild portal hypertension MR images show dilation of the portal vein, and possibly splenic vein. In more severe and chronic cases, the portal vein can occlude and become thin or unapparent, with development of multiple smaller-caliber collaterals seen within the portahepatis, so-called "cavernous transformation." Furthermore, portosystemic collaterals can form and be seen as increased number and size of retroperitoneal vessels in the region of the splenic hilum, gastrohepatic ligament, paraesophageal region (Fig. 16), and with demonstration of splenorenal venous connections. Canalization of the periumbilical vein can be seen as a vessel, sometimes massive, extending from the left portal vein anteriorly along the falciform ligament toward the anterior abdominal wall umbilical region (see Fig. 16). Ascites is commonly seen in combination with more advanced portal hypertension as simple uniform high signal T2-weighted fluid in the free intraperitoneal space.

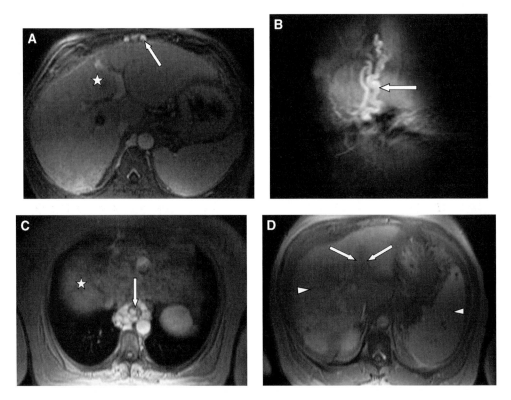

Fig. 16. Venous abnormalities related to cirrhosis in three different patients. Axial T1-weighted breathhold SGE fat-suppressed postgadolinium delayed phase (A) and coronal (B) images show recanalized periumbilical vein (arrow), arising from the left portal vein (A, arrow), and extending to the anterior midline peritoneum. A mass representing HCC is present (star). In a second case (C), advanced coarse linear and reticular hepatic fibrosis is shown with late enhancement (star). There are prominent varices encasing and lifting the distal esophagus (arrow) in this patient with esophageal hemorrhage. On a third case (D), the left portal vein (arrows) is markedly distended with enhancing soft tissue in this patient with HCC and portal vein tumor thrombus. The arrowheads indicate siderotic nodules in the liver and spleen.

Budd-Chiari (hepatic vein thrombosis)

The original description of Budd-Chiari syndrome related to a severe, often fatal, acute form of hepatic vein thrombosis [53]. Currently, Budd-Chiari is used to describe any form of pathology related to hepatic venous thrombosis [53]. Thrombosis within hepatic veins most commonly occurs as a result of hyper-coagulable states; occurs more commonly in women; and can be associated with underlying conditions including pregnancy or postpartum state, lupus, sepsis, polycythemia, and neoplasm, particularly HCC.

In Budd-Chiari, hepatic venous outflow obstruction results in congestion and ischemia, which over

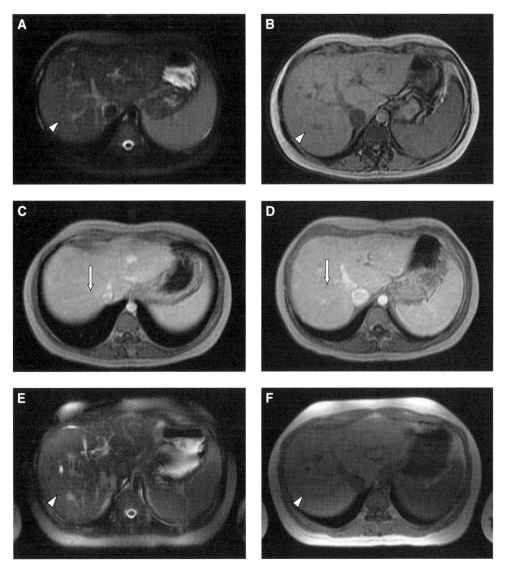

Fig. 17. Budd-Chiari syndrome with hepatic segmental venous thrombosis imaged acutely (*A–D*) and after 6 months (*E* and *F*). Axial images of the liver (*A–F*) show abnormal elevated signal on T2-weighted breathhold single shot fast spin echo imaging (*A*) in the right lobe (*A, arrowhead*), with corresponding diminished signal on T1-weighted unenhanced breathhold SGE (*B, arrowhead*). Venous-phase gadolinium-enhanced images at two levels (*C* and *D*) demonstrate a thrombosed segmental branch of the right hepatic vein (*arrow*). Follow-up imaging in the subacute-chronic stages shows diminishment in the elevated signal on T2-weighted imaging (*E* versus *A, arrowhead*), and restoration of T1-weighted signal (*F* versus *B, arrowhead*). There is development of abnormal patchy increased peripheral enhancement on the arterial phase image (*G, arrowhead*) becoming more uniform on venous phase (*H*). The thrombosed vessel (*C* and *D, arrow*) has become unapparent (*H* versus *C, arrow*).

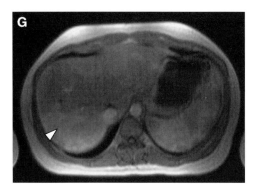 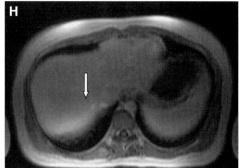

Fig. 17 (*continued*).

time can lead to atrophy and fibrosis [53]. Depending on degree of involvement, relatively spared segments of liver undergo compensatory hypertrophy. The caudate lobe characteristically has separate drainage to the inferior vena cava and is usually spared, and commonly can be seen to hypertrophy over time [53]. Hepatic venous drainage is quite variable, and other segments of liver are commonly spared, leading to variable regions of hypertrophy.

The characteristic liver MR imaging pattern (Fig. 17) of Budd-Chiari in the acute, subacute, and chronic states has been described [53]. In the acute state, central liver shows low T1-, and mildly elevated T2-weighted signal secondary to edema, with irregular increased enhancement in the arterial postgadolinium phase images [53]. In the subacute phase, this pattern of T1- and T2-weighted signal intensity and postgadolinium enhancement is seen to migrate toward the periphery of the liver [53]. In both acute and subacute states, hepatic vein thrombosis is best visualized on postgadolinium venous or delayed-phase breathhold SGE images (see Fig. 16). In the chronic phase, visualization of the hepatic vein thrombus may become less apparent; however, there is a characteristic hypertrophy of the caudate lobe, often massive, and hypertrophy of other spared segments [53]. The liver segments affected by chronic hepatic venous obstruction show atrophy and fibrosis. Fibrotic regions may show progressively increasing enhancement on delayed postgadolinium images, with regenerative nodules showing relatively higher T1-weighted signal, and intermediate to low T2-weighted signal, with marked enhancement on arterial-venous phase postgadolinium SGE images.

When hepatic venous thrombosis results from direct invasion by tumor, this is most commonly related to HCC. In the case of tumor thrombosis, demonstration of soft tissue enhancement on post-gadolinium breathhold T1-weighted SGE images is diagnostic.

References

[1] Brenner DJ, Elliston CD. Estimated radiation risks potentially associated with full body CT screening. Radiology 2004;232:735–8.

[2] Gleeson TG, Bulugahapitiya S. Contrast-induced nephropathy. AJR Am J Roentgenol 2004;183:1673–89.

[3] Harkonen S, Kjellstrand CM. Exacerbation of diabetic renal failure following intravenous pyelography. Am J Med 1977;63:939–46.

[4] Manske CL, Sprafka JM, Storry JT, et al. Contrast nephropathy in azotemicdiabetic patients undergoing coronary angiography. Am J Med 1990;89:615–20.

[5] Gaa J, Hutabu H, Jenkins RL, et al. Liver masses: replacement of conventional T2-weighted spin echo MR imaging with breath-hold MR imaging. Radiology 1996;200:459–64.

[6] Bradley WG. Optimizing lesion contrast without using contrast agents. J Magn Reson Imaging 1999; 10:442–9.

[7] Coates GG, Borrello JA, McFarland EG, et al. Hepatic T2-weighted MRI: a prospective comparison of sequences, including breath-hold, half-Fourier turbo spin echo (HASTE). J Magn Reson Imaging 1998;8: 642–9.

[8] Helmberger TK, Schroder J, Holzknecht N, et al. T2-weighted breathhold imaging of the liver: a quantitative and qualitative comparison of fast spin echo and half Fourier single shot fast spin echo imaging. MAGMA 1999;9:42–51.

[9] Semelka RC, Martin DR, Balci C, et al. Focal liver lesions: comparison of dual-phase CT and multi-sequence multiplanar MR imaging including dynamic gadolinium enhancement. J Magn Reson Imaging 2001;13:397–401.

[10] Martin DR, Semelka RC, Chung JJ, et al. Sequential use of gadolinium chelate and mangafodipir triso-

dium for the assessment of focal liver lesions: initial observations. Magn Reson Imaging 2000;18:955 – 63.

[11] Naganawa S, Jenner G, Cooper TG, et al. Rapid MR imaging of the liver: comparison of twelve techniques for single breath-hold whole volume acquisition. Radiat Med 1994;12:255 – 61.

[12] Semelka RC, Kelekis NL, Thomasson D, et al. HASTE MR imaging: description of technique and preliminary results in the abdomen. J Magn Reson Imaging 1996;6:698 – 9.

[13] Semelka RC, Balci NC, Op de Beeck B, et al. Evaluation of a 10-minute comprehensive MR imaging examination of the upper abdomen. Radiology 1999; 211:189 – 95.

[14] Siewert B, Muller MF, Foley M, et al. Fast MR imaging of the liver: quantitative comparison of techniques. Radiology 1994;193:37 – 42.

[15] Chien D, Edelman RR. Ultrafast imaging using gradient echoes. Magn Reson Q 1991;7:31 – 56.

[16] Rofsky NM, Lee VS, Laub G, et al. Abdominal MR imaging with a volumetric interpolated breath-hold examination. Radiology 1999;212:876 – 84.

[17] Semelka RC, Brown ED, Ascher SM, et al. Hepatic hemangiomas: a multi-institutional study of appearance on T2- weighted and serial gadolinium-enhanced gradient-echo MR images. Radiology 1994; 192:401 – 6.

[18] Kelekis NL, Semelka RC, Worawattanakul S, et al. Hepatocellular carcinoma in North America: a multi-institutional study of appearance on T1-weighted, T2-weighted, and serial gadolinium- enhanced gradient-echo images. AJR Am J Roentgenol 1998;170:1005 – 13.

[19] Imam K, Bluemke DA. MR imaging in the evaluation of hepatic metastases. Magn Reson Imaging Clin N Am 2000;8:741 – 56.

[20] Larson RE, Semelka RC, Bagley AS, et al. Hypervascular malignant liver lesions: comparison of various MR imaging pulse sequences and dynamic CT. Radiology 1994;192:393 – 9.

[21] Low RN. Current uses of gadolinium chelates for clinical magnetic resonance imaging examination of the liver. Top Magn Reson Imaging 1998;9:141 – 66.

[22] Reimer P, Rummeny EJ, Daldrup HE, et al. Enhancement characteristics of liver metastases, hepatocellular carcinomas, and hemangiomas with Gd-EOB-DTPA: preliminary results with dynamic MR imaging. Eur Radiol 1997;7:275 – 80.

[23] Imai Y, Murakami T, Yoshida S, et al. Superparamagnetic iron oxide-enhanced magnetic resonance images of hepatocellular carcinoma: correlation with histological grading. Hepatology 2000;32:205 – 12.

[24] Muller RD, Vogel K, Neumann K, et al. SPIO-MR imaging versus double-phase spiral CT in detecting malignant lesions of the liver. Acta Radiol 1999;40: 628 – 35.

[25] Ferrucci JT. Advances in abdominal MR imaging. Radiographics 1998;18:1569 – 86.

[26] Semelka RC, Lee JK, Worawattanakul S, et al. Sequential use of ferumoxide particles and gadolinium chelate for the evaluation of focal liver lesions on MRI. J Magn Reson Imaging 1998;8:670 – 4.

[27] Ni Y, Marchal G. Enhanced magnetic resonance imaging for tissue characterization of liver abnormalities with hepatobiliary contrast agents: an overview of preclinical animal experiments. Top Magn Reson Imaging 1998;9:183 – 95.

[28] Torres CG, Lundby B, Sterud AT, et al. MnDPDP for MR imaging of the liver: results from the European phase III studies. Acta Radiol 1997;38:631 – 7.

[29] Fretz CJ, Stark DD, Metz CE, et al. Detection of hepatic metastases: comparison of contrast-enhanced CT, unenhanced MR imaging, and iron oxide-enhanced MR imaging. AJR Am J Roentgenol 1990; 155:763 – 70.

[30] Schmidt AJ, Kee ST, Sze DY, et al. Diagnostic yield of MR-guided liver biopsies compared with CT- and US-guided liver biopsies. J Vasc Interv Radiol 1999; 10:1323 – 9.

[31] Braga L, Semelka RC, Pietrobon R, et al. Does hypervascularity of liver metastases as detected on MRI predict disease progression in breast cancer patients? AJR Am J Roentgenol 2004;182:1207 – 13.

[32] Siegelman ES. MR imaging of diffuse liver disease: hepatic fat and iron. Magn Reson Imaging Clin N Am 1997;5:347 – 65.

[33] Thu HD, Mathieu D, Thu NT, et al. Value of MR imaging in evaluating focal fatty infiltration of the liver: preliminary study. Radiographics 1991;11:1003 – 12.

[34] Rofsky NM, Weinreb JC, Ambrosino MM, et al. Comparison between in-phase and opposed-phase T1-weighted breath-hold FLASH sequences for hepatic imaging. J Comput Assist Tomogr 1996;20:230 – 5.

[35] Kier R, Mason BJ. Water-suppressed MR imaging of focal fatty infiltration of the liver. Radiology 1997; 203:575 – 7.

[36] Mitchell DG. Chemical shift magnetic resonance imaging: applications in the abdomen and pelvis. Top Magn Reson Imaging 1992;4:46 – 63.

[37] Siegelman ES, Mitchell DG, Semelka RC. Abdominal iron deposition: metabolism, MR findings, and clinical importance. Radiology 1996;199:13 – 22.

[38] Thomsen C, Wiggers P, Ring-Larsen H, et al. Identification of patients with hereditary haemochromatosis by magnetic resonance imaging and spectroscopic relaxation time measurements. Magn Reson Imaging 1992;10:867 – 79.

[39] Engelhardt R, Langkowski JH, Fischer R, et al. Liver iron quantification: studies in aqueous iron solutions, iron overloaded rats, and patients with hereditary hemochromatosis. Magn Reson Imaging 1994;12:999 – 1007.

[40] Gandon Y, Guyader D, Heautot JF, et al. Hemochromatosis: diagnosis and quantification of liver iron with gradient-echo MR imaging. Radiology 1994;193: 533 – 8.

[41] Keevil SF, Alstead EM, Dolke G, et al. Non-invasive assessment of diffuse liver disease by in vivo measurement of proton nuclear magnetic resonance relaxation times at 0.08 T. Br J Radiol 1994;67:1083 – 7.

[42] Bonetti MG, Castriota-Scanderbeg A, Criconia GM, et al. Hepatic iron overload in thalassemic patients: proposal and validation of an MRI method of assessment. Pediatr Radiol 1996;26:650–6.

[43] Ernst O, Sergent G, Bonvarlet P, et al. Hepatic iron overload: diagnosis and quantification with MR imaging. AJR Am J Roentgenol 1997;168:1205–8.

[44] Gandon Y, Olivie D, Guyader D. Non-invasive assessment of hepatic iron stores by MRI. Lancet 2004; 363:357–62.

[45] Alustiza JM, Artetxe J, Castiella A. MR quantification of hepatic iron concentration. Radiology 2004;230: 479–84.

[46] Semelka RC, Chung JJ, Hussain SM, et al. Chronic hepatitis: correlation of early patchy and late linear enhancement patterns on gadolinium-enhanced MR images with histopathology initial experience. J Magn Reson Imaging 2001;13:385–91.

[47] Matsui O, Kadoya M, Takashima T, et al. Intrahepatic periportal abnormal intensity on MR images: an indication of various hepatobiliary diseases. Radiology 1989;171:335–8.

[48] Marzola P, Maggioni F, Vicinanza E, et al. Evaluation of the hepatocyte-specific contrast agent gadobenate dimeglumine for MR imaging of acute hepatitis in a rat model. J Magn Reson Imaging 1997;7:147–52.

[49] Martin DR, Seibert D, Yang M, et al. Reversible heterogeneous arterial phase liver perfusion. associated with transient acute hepatitis: findings on gadolinium-enhanced MRI. J Magn Reson Imaging 2004;20: 838–42.

[50] Kreft B, Dombrowski F, Block W, et al. Evaluation of different models of experimentally induced liver cirrhosis for MRI research with correlation to histopathologic findings. Invest Radiol 1999;34:360–6.

[51] King LJ, Scurr ED, Murugan N, et al. Hepatobiliary and pancreatic manifestations of cystic fibrosis: MR imaging appearances. Radiographics 2000;20:767–77.

[52] Koolpe HA, Koolpe L. Portal hypertension: angiographic and hemodynamic evaluation. Radiol Clin North Am 1986;24:369–81.

[53] Noone TC, Semelka RC, Siegelman ES, et al. Budd-Chiari syndrome: spectrum of appearances of acute, subacute, and chronic disease with magnetic resonance imaging. J Magn Reson Imaging 2000;11:44–50.

RADIOLOGIC CLINICS of North America

Radiol Clin N Am 43 (2005) 887–898

Contrast Agents for MR Imaging of the Liver

N. Cem Balci, MD[a],*, Richard C. Semelka, MD[b]

[a]Department of Radiology, Saint Louis University, St. Louis, MO, USA
[b]Department of Radiology, School of Medicine, University of North Carolina, Chapel Hill, NC, USA

Imaging of the liver is performed most often to detect and characterize focal liver lesions. MR imaging has been the method of choice to assess focal liver lesions accurately. Nonspecific intravenous contrast agents have been used for routine abdominal MR imaging protocols including liver imaging. These agents are distributed in the extracellular space, and have comparable imaging hemodynamics as extracellular contrast agents used in CT, even though their mechanism of action is completely different. Although gadolinium (Gd)-chelate compounds generally evoke the same perfusion-related tissue characteristic seen with contrast-enhanced CT, there is superior tissue contrast in MR imaging.

Over the last 10 to 15 years new contrast agents have been developed that combine the excellent contrast resolution of MR imaging with improved tissue specificity. Intravenously administered liver-specific contrast agents are either selectively taken up by hepatocytes or by the reticuloendothelial system in the liver (Kupffer cells). Some of these agents also have the combined properties of an extracellular contrast agent and selective tissue uptake. This article reviews various contrast agents that are in clinical use for liver MR imaging and discusses their potential clinical role.

Nonspecific extracellular contrast agents

The nonspecific contrast agents with extracellular biodistribution are Gd-chelates. A variety of Gd-chelates are produced with different binding complexes that behave similarly. Free Gd is toxic in vivo and forms colloid particles that are phagocytized by the reticuloendothelial system. The binding to a chelate complex makes the ion chemically inert [1–3]. The list of contrast agents used for abdominal and hepatic MR imaging includes different Gd-chelates with their corresponding brand names (Table 1). Gd-chelates are used with a standard dose of 0.1 mmol/kg for abdominal imaging. Most of the Gd-chelates result in minor changes in the serum iron and bilirubin levels and demonstrate passage across the placenta and excretion into the breast milk [4]. This occurs within 24 hours of injection. The use of Gd-chelates during pregnancy or breast-feeding is generally not recommended, but they can be used if clinically important. Adverse reactions are observed with an incidence of less than 2%, with most being mild and transient. Anaphylactoid reactions have been reported [1,3].

Gd-chelates are distributed in the abdomen in the intravascular and interstitial spaces. After intravenous injection, Gd-chelates follow the route of blood circulation in the body. In the abdomen, the contrast agent first reaches the aorta and its branches. Contrast enters the splanchnic and splenic circulation by the celiac axis, superior and inferior mesenteric arteries, and then into their companion veins and subsequently into the portal vein. Contrast agent enters the venous system after the passage through the sinusoids in the liver, and after passing the capillaries in the pe-

* Corresponding author. Department of Radiology, Saint Louis University, 3635 Vista Avenue, DT-2, St. Louis, MO.
E-mail address: nc.balci@excite.com (N.C. Balci).

Table 1
Extracellular contrast agents for abdominal and hepatic MR imaging

Acronym	Generic name	Brand name	Companies (location)
Gd-DTPA	Gadopentetate dimeglumine	Magnevist	Schering AG (Berlin, Germany); Berlex Laboratories (Montville, NJ)
Gd-DOTA	Gadoterate meglumine	Dotarem	Guerbet (Aulney-sous-Bois, France)
Gd-DTPA-BMA	Gadodiamide	Omniscan	Nycomed Amersham (Oslo, Norway)
Gd-HP-DO3A	Gadoteridol	ProHance	Bracco SpA (Milan, Italy)
Gd-DTPA-bis-methoxyethylamide	Gadoversetamide	OptiMARK	Mallinckrodt Medical (St. Louis, MO)

ripheral circulation. The temporal enhancement pattern of the liver and any focal lesions determine the detection and characterization of focal and diffuse liver pathologies. Imaging with increased temporal resolution including bolus injection of the contrast agent is required. The recommended injection rate of these contrast agents is 2 to 3 mL/s. The serial contrast-enhanced images are acquired with the use of T1-weighted gradient echo sequences, either two- or three-dimensional [1,3].

Hepatic imaging with nonspecific extracellular contrast agents is performed mainly in three consecutive temporal phases related to the location of the bulk of the contrast agent in the abdomen and the liver: the central phase-encoding step of the hepatic arterial-dominant phase is approximately 28 seconds after the initiation of bolus injection of the contrast agent. In this phase, contrast enhancement is observed in the hepatic artery and portal vein, and not in the hepatic veins. Hepatic parenchyma is mildly

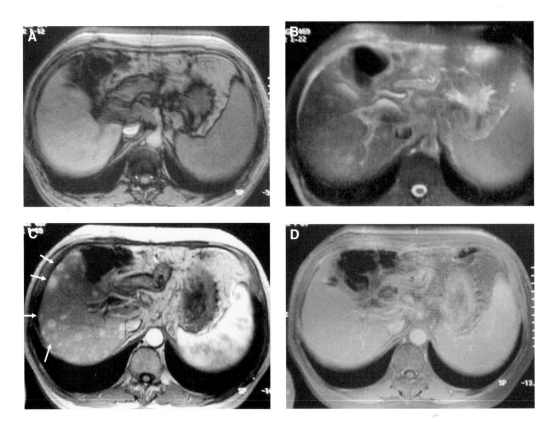

Fig. 1. Serial contrast-enhanced MR image of the liver in a patient with hypervascular liver metastases. (*A*) T1-weighted spoiled gradient echo image in axial plane reveals no focal liver lesions. (*B*) On T2-weighted fat-saturated single shot echo train image in axial plane, there are no visible focal liver lesions. (*C*) On arterial-phase serial contrast-enhanced images multiple hypervascular metastases are demonstrated (*arrows*). (*D*) On late-phase serial contrast-enhanced images, these lesions fade and are not visible.

enhanced. During this phase, other abdominal organs with rich capillary blood supply, such as the kidneys and the pancreas, reveal contrast enhancement. During the hepatic-arterial phase hypervascular liver pathologies are depicted and characterized (Fig. 1). Portal-venous phase (early hepatic-venous phase) is approximately 1 minute after the initiation of the contrast injection. During this phase contrast enhancement in the hepatic veins is observed and hepatic parenchyma is nearly maximally enhanced. Maximal vascular opacification is observed in this phase. Assessment of hypovascular liver pathologies and washout of hypervascular pathologies also occur in this phase. Late hepatic-venous or interstitial phase is the time interval approximately 90 seconds to 5 minutes after initiation of contrast injection. During this phase of enhancement hepatic parenchymal enhancement persists. This phase provides additional information further to characterize focal hepatic lesions, by demonstrating their late-phase temporal handling of contrast. Hemangiomas reveal progressive enhancement, persistent enhancement is observed in small-sized hemangiomas, and washout of hypervascular metastases and HCC is also apparent during this phase [1].

Serial contrast-enhanced imaging with the use of nonspecific extracellular contrast agents has high accuracy in detecting and characterizing focal liver lesions. In some focal liver lesions, such as hepatocellular carcinoma (HCC), focal nodular hyperplasia (FNH), and adenomas, the enhancement pattern may not be confident for the differential diagnosis between lesions of liver origin and malignant lesions. Liver-specific contrast agents may play a role [5–9].

Liver-specific contrast agents

Liver-specific contrast agents make up a group of contrast agents that reveal intracellular uptake by cells located in the liver. According to the hepatic cells that show uptake, they are divided into two groups: hepatocyte-selective and Kupffer cell–specific contrast agents.

Hepatocyte-selective agents are either only hepatocyte selective, such as mangafodipir trisodium (Mn-DPDP; Amersham, Oslo, Norway), or are Gd-chelates (gadobenate dimeglumine [Gd-BOPTA; Bracco, Milan, Italy] and Gd-ethoxybenzyl [Gd-EOB; Schering AG, Berlin, Germany]) that are both distributed in the extracellular space and are hepatocyte selective. Kupffer cell–specific contrast agents are iron-containing compounds. The hepatocyte-specific Gd-chelates and Mn-DPDP are T1 agents, which shorten T1 time and result in increased signal on T1-weighted images. Kupffer cell–specific agents shorten T2 and T1 times, with a predominant effect of decreasing T2 signal, but with increase of T1 signal in some settings.

Hepatocyte-selective contrast agents

Mangafodipir trisodium

Mn-DPDP is an anionic manganese chelate that dissociates rapidly following administration yielding free Mn^{++} ion. Free Mn^{++} is taken up by the hepatocytes and eliminated by the hepatobiliary pathway, and also shows uptake by the renal cortex, pancreas, and gastric mucosa. Free Mn^{++} may cause an increased neurologic risk in patients with hepatic impairment. Mn-DPDP shortens the T1 time and causes increased signal in the liver on T1-weighted images [10–12]. T1-weighted breathhold gradient echo sequences are well suited for image acquisition. A T1-weighted spin echo sequence may be used in patients who have difficulty in holding their breath. Mn-DPDP is administered as a slow intravenous infusion over 1 to 2 minutes with a dose of 5 μmol/kg. Maximum liver enhancement is observed within 10 to 15 minutes after the infusion. After slow-drip infusion, facial flushing and perception of increased body temperature may occur as a reported side effect. Serious side effects have not been described [10–12]. On postcontrast images, lesions without hepatocyte content remain unenhanced including metastases, benign liver cysts, and hemangiomas. Most tumors of nonhepatocellular origin typically are hypointense relative to enhanced liver parenchyma on T1-weighted images and are more conspicuous than on unenhanced images (Fig. 2). Tumors of hepatocellular origin, such as FNH, adenoma, and well-differentiated HCC, have been shown to accumulate Mn-DPDP, providing characterization information to discriminate hepatocellular from nonhepatocellular tumors. Although Mn-DPDP can differentiate between hepatocyte- and non–hepatocyte-containing lesions, it may not be that effective in the differentiation between benign and malignant lesions. Regenerating nodules, well-differentiated HCC, and metastases from endocrine tumors reveal contrast uptake and increased enhancement. Benign and malignant hepatocellular tumors reveal varying degrees of enhancement that can be observed up to 24 hours after administration [13–15].

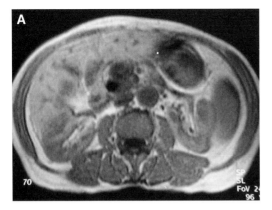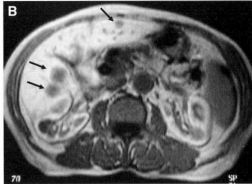

Fig. 2. Liver metastases from pancreatic adenocarcinoma. (*A*) On T1-weighted spoiled gradient echo image before administration of Mn-DPDP, the metastatic lesions cannot be delineated. (*B*) After application of intravenous Mn-DPDP three liver metastases were depicted (*arrows*).

Gadobenate dimeglumine

Gd-BOPTA combines the properties of a conventional nonspecific Gd agent with that of a hepatocyte-selective agent. Gd-BOPTA is an octadentate chelate of the paramagnetic ion Gd. This agent differs from other available Gd-chelates in that it distributes not only to the extracellular fluid space, but is selectively taken up by functioning hepatocytes and excreted into the bile by the canalicular multispecific organic anion transporter that is used to eliminate bilirubin [16–18]. Gd-BOPTA is mainly eliminated by the kidneys. Although the biliary excretion rate is 55% in rats and 25% in rabbits, respectively, it is only 3% to 5% in humans [19]. This agent results in prolonged enhancement of the liver parenchyma combined with the plasma kinetics of an extracellular agent. The hepatobiliary contrast enhancement is most promi-

nent 60 to 120 minutes after intravenous injection. The liver parenchyma enhancement obtained with Gd-BOPTA is comparable with the enhancement level of purely liver-specific contrast media [20]. Gd-BOPTA has a higher relaxivity than equimolar formulations of other approved extracellular contrast agents, such as gadopentetate dimeglumine (Schering AG, Berlin, Germany), gadodiamide (Amersham-Health, Oslo, Norway), and gadoterate meglumine (Guerbet, Aulnay-sous-Bois, France) [21], because of its more lipophilic structure and its capacity for weak and transient interaction with serum albumin (Fig. 3) [22]. In the liver, the estimated relaxivity is about 30 $\text{mmol}^{-1} \text{ s}^{-1}$, compared with calculated values of 16.6 $\text{mmol}^{-1} \text{ s}^{-1}$ for Gd-ethoxybenzyl–diethylenetriamine pentaacetic acid (Gd-EOB-DTPA) and 21.7 $\text{mmol}^{-1} \text{ s}^{-1}$ for Mn-DPDP [23]. This effect is thought to be caused more by increased intra-

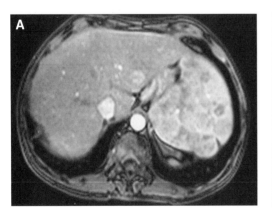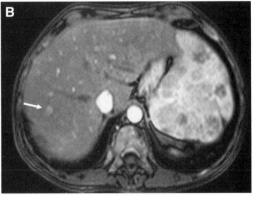

Fig. 3. Hypervascular liver metastasis from renal cell carcinoma. (*A*) On T1-weighted spoiled gradient echo image in arterial phase with 0.1 mmol/kg, Gd-DTPA reveals no focal liver lesion. (*B*) Same patient is examined with 0.1 mmol/kg Gd-BOPTA, which depicts the hypervascular metastasis in the anterior segment of the right liver lobe (*arrow*).

cellular microviscosity within the hepatocytes than by transient interactions with intracellular proteins [24]. Gd-BOPTA has been approved in many European countries for MR imaging of the liver since 1998; up to 2001 this contrast agent has been administered to about 100,000 patients. This clinical experience has shown that Gd-BOPTA is well tolerated, even in patients with moderate to severe renal failure. This agent has recently been approved for use in the United States.

Serial contrast-enhanced liver imaging can be performed with the use of Gd-BOPTA after bolus injection (see Fig. 3), in the same fashion as with other nonspecific extracellular contrast agents [10]. Serial contrast-enhanced images exploit the differences in blood supply between lesions and normal liver parenchyma. The results are comparable with other conventional extracellular contrast agents, particularly for the improved visualization of hypervascular lesions (Figs. 3 and 4) [10]. Furthermore, Gd-BOPTA, similar to other extracellular contrast agents, allows improved assessment of lesion hemodynamics [10,25–28]. Improvement in the detection of hypovascular lesions has also been reported with Gd-BOPTA compared with standard extracellular agents [10,29]. This reflects the fact that an increased fraction of Gd-BOPTA is taken up by the hepatocytes, which translates into increased detection and delineation of hypovascular lesions on delayed (40–120 min postinjection) or static hepatobiliary liver imaging (see Fig. 4). Uptake of Gd-BOPTA may be relatively increased in cirrhotic as compared with noncirrhotic liver parenchyma. Uptake of the agent into regenerative nodules and well-differentiated HCC is observed. Kuwatsuru and coworkers [30] compared Gd-BOPTA with gadopentetate dimeglumine in 257 patients suspected of having malignant liver tumors [10] and they observed that the contrast efficacy on early dynamic postcontrast images was comparable, whereas on delayed images Gd-BOPTA was significantly superior to gadopentetate dimeglumine in terms of improvement over the nonenhanced scans (44.5% versus 19% on breathhold gradient echo sequences).

In a multicenter, multireader study involving 214 patients, Petersein and coworkers [31] reported a significantly increased number of lesions detected on delayed postcontrast images. Furthermore, the average size of detected lesions was smaller, reflecting improved depiction of small lesions, whereas the conspicuity of all lesions improved. All on-site readers and two of three off-site readers reported an increase in overall diagnostic confidence. In addition, further information on lesion characterization was provided in up to 25% of dynamic-phase images and 59% of delayed-phase postcontrast images, compared with the noncontrast scans [10]. Schneider and coworkers [32] similarly reported a tendency toward more accurate results after Gd-BOPTA than after gadopentetate dimeglumine in a study of 43 patients. Morana and coworkers [33] examined 249 patients with a variety of primary and secondary hypervascular tumors on both dynamic and delayed imaging. They found that delayed imaging gave additional information for lesion characterization with high accuracy in distinguishing benign lesions like FNH and regenerative hyperplasia from other lesion types (sensitivity 79.7%, specificity 96.1%). Grazioli and coworkers [34] studied a subset of patients with FNH comparing Gd-BOPTA with ferumoxides. They noted

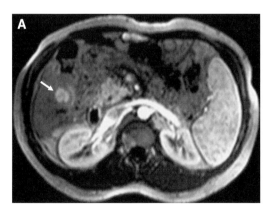 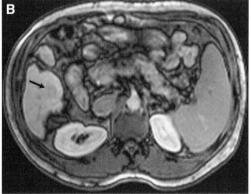

Fig. 4. HCC in a cirrhotic liver. (A) Arterial-phase serial contrast-enhanced spoiled gradient echo image with the use of Gd-BOPTA reveals a focal liver lesion with prominent arterial enhancement. (B) The same lesion reveals diminished enhancement in the late hepatobiliary phase (arrow), because of the small number of hepatocytes in the lesion.

that 57 of 60 lesions displayed typical enhancement characteristics after Gd-BOPTA and 100% were identified correctly, whereas after ferumoxides only 27 of 43 lesions showed typical enhancement, with 71.6% correctly identified as FNH. Differentiation between hepatocellular adenomas and FNH is possible with the use of Gd-BOPTA during the hepatobiliary phase. FNH contains biliary ducts, whereas hepatocellular adenoma does not have biliary ducts. In the hepatobiliary phase FNH reveals increased enhancement as compared with hepatocellular adenomas (Fig. 5). Gd-BOPTA is an effective extracellular contrast agent. The greater T1 relaxivity allows better visualization of hypervascular lesions compared with conventional extracellular agents and equivalent lesion detection when used in half dose. The hepatocyte selectivity further helps to distinguish hepatocyte-containing lesions from other focal liver lesions. Long waiting time for the hepatobiliary phase imaging, however, may be a disadvantage in daily practice.

Gadolinium-ethoxybenzyl–diethylenetriamine pentaacetic-acid

Gd-EOB-DTPA is a paramagnetic hepatobiliary contrast agent with hepatocellular uptake by the anionic-transporter protein [35,36]. Gd-EOB-DTPA has higher T1-relaxivity in human plasma ($R1$ 8.2 $mmol^{-1}$ s^{-1}) than gadopentetate dimeglumine ($R1$ 5 $mmol^{-1}$ s^{-1}). This may be explained by the greater degree of protein binding compared with gadopentetate dimeglumine. Gd-EOB-DTPA provides a triphasic pharmacokinetic profile similar to that of Gd-BOPTA. The lipophilic side chain EOB produces a high affinity to the organic anion transporter system, which is also responsible for the uptake of Gd-BOPTA. After intravenous bolus injection, Gd-EOB-DTPA is rapidly cleared from the intravascular space to the extracellular space; from here the compound is both taken up by hepatocytes and eliminated by glomerular filtration. In contrast to

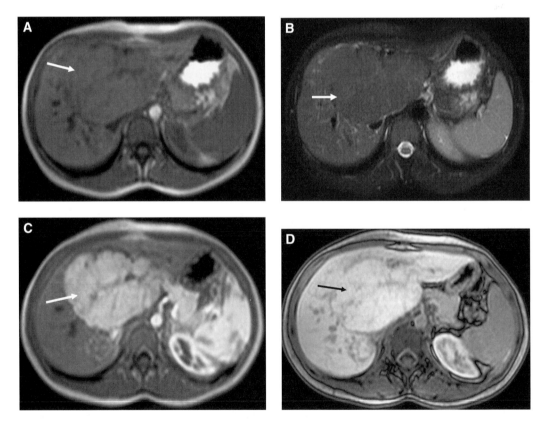

Fig. 5. Giant FNH in the left liver lobe. On T1-weighted spoiled gradient echo image (*A*) and on T2-weighted fat-saturated echo train image (*B*), the lesion is isointense with the liver parenchyma (*arrow*). On arterial phase T1-weighted spoiled gradient echo image after Gd-BOPTA (*C*), the lesion reveals prominent enhancement (*arrow*), which reveals persistent contrast enhancement during late hepatobiliary phase (*D*) consistent with the hepatocyte and biliary duct content of FNH.

Gd-BOPTA, urinary filtration and fecal excretion by way of bile fluid account for approximately equal portions of the administered dose. Although the degree of renal elimination rises with increasing doses, its hepatic clearance reveals a moderate saturation phenomenon in higher doses.

Hepatobiliary contrast enhancement with Gd-EOB-DTPA reaches the maximum level at about 10 to 20 minutes postinjection and is followed by a plateau phase that has duration of 2 hours. The highest liver-to-lesion contrast is observed during the imaging window 20 to 45 minutes after injection of Gd-EOB-DTPA, as compared with 60 to 120 minutes postinjection period for delayed-phase imaging with Gd-BOPTA.

In phase 1 studies, the safety and pharmacokinetics of Gd-EOB-DTPA was tested at doses of 10, 25, 50, and 100 μmol Gd/kg of body weight. Results of laboratory tests, clinical measurements, and pharmacokinetic data were obtained in 44 healthy volunteers in a double-blinded, randomized, and placebo-controlled design. Gd-EOB-DTPA was well tolerated, with no important side effects or changes in laboratory parameters [37]. During subsequent clinical phase 2 trials, the diagnostic efficacy and safety of Gd-EOB-DTPA was explored at five doses (3, 6, 12.5, 25, and 50 μmol Gd-EOB-DTPA/kg body weight) as compared with the placebo (0.9% saline) in patients with known focal liver lesions. Safety variables included evaluation of vital signs, physical examination, clinical laboratory tests, and adverse events. A total of 171 received contrast medium injection or placebo (0.9% saline) in phase 2B (87 men and 84 women, age range 26–82 years, median age 59 years for men and 57 years for women). No serious adverse events were reported in any of the patients. In six patients eight adverse events were seen without dose dependency. Of these four adverse events, 4% were considered as possibly or probably drug related. All adverse events were mild except one case of anxiety. No significant changes in vital signs or laboratory parameters were observed [38,39]. Within the subsequent phase 3 multicenter trial, no clinically relevant changes in hemodynamic or laboratory parameters were observed. Of the 162 patients who received Gd-EOB-DTPA injection, a total of 11 patients (6.8%) reported 21 adverse effects independent of drug relationship. The most frequently reported symptoms of definitely, possibly, or probably related adverse effects were nausea, vasodilatation, headache, taste perversion, and injection site pain [38].

A phase 2 study investigated the dose-dependent diagnostic efficacy of Gd-EOB-DTPA. Doses of 12.5, 25, or 50 μmol Gd-EOB-DTPA/kg body weight (corresponding to injection volumes of 3.5, 7, and 14 mL in a 70-kg patient) were studied within the format of a double-blind and randomized dose-ranging clinical trial. This multicenter trial revealed no significant differences both for lesion detection and characterization among the previously mentioned three doses tested [38]. In a second dose-finding multicenter, double-blind, randomized, and placebo-controlled dose-ranging study [39] the diagnostic efficacy and safety of Gd-EOB-DTPA at four doses (3, 6, 12.5, and 25 μmol Gd-EOB-DTPA/kg) was investigated in 171 patients with known focal liver lesions. The efficacy assessment included lesion detection, classification and characterization, signal-to-noise ratio, contrast-to-noise ratio, percent enhancement, visual evaluation of lesions, impact on patient management, and diagnostic confidence. Improved lesion visualization and delineation was observed in dose groups of 6, 12.5, and 25 μmol/kg. Increased enhancement of hepatic vessels and liver parenchyma during dynamic imaging was observed with the higher doses. A dose-dependent increase in signal-to-noise ratio, contrast-to-noise ratio, and relative enhancement was reported, which was most pronounced at 25 μmol/kg. Diagnostic efficacy did not change at 45 minutes postinjection compared with 20 minutes postinjection [39]. As a result of this phase 2B study 25 μmol/kg was considered the optimum dose [39].

The diagnostic performance of Gd-EOB-DTPA–enhanced MR imaging for detection of liver lesions was evaluated in a prospective, open-label, within-patient comparison phase 3 study with the use of 25 μmol/kg dose [40]. Acquired images were assessed during early phase serial contrast-enhanced imaging and hepatobiliary late-phase imaging. A total of 302 histopathologically or intraoperative ultrasound-verified lesions in 131 patients were evaluated. Among the lesions, 215 were malignant, 80 were benign, and 7 lesions were not assessable. The malignant lesions were metastases (N = 172); HCC (N = 31); and cholangiocellular carcinomas (N = 12). The benign lesions included 41 liver cysts; 18 hemangiomas; 7 FNH; and 14 other benign lesions (adenomas, hydatid cysts, abscesses, and so forth). The percentage of correctly matched lesions increased from 80.8% on precontrast MR imaging to 87.4% on postcontrast MR imaging. The correct classification of lesions also improved significantly. In the off-site reading, as in the clinical on-site study, more small lesions were detected on postcontrast than on precontrast images.

Hypervascular metastatic lesions revealed their most prominent enhancement in the early arterial phase, whereas hypovascular metastases showed highest enhancement 90 to 120 seconds following intravenous injection of Gd-EOB-DTPA, then gradually decreased and stabilized >10 minutes following contrast injection. HCC demonstrated increased enhancement in the initial distribution phase 60 seconds following intravenous injection of Gd-EOB-DTPA similar to liver parenchyma, with more prolonged enhancement compared with metastases and liver parenchyma, and enhancement of HCC was similar during the complete observation period. Following increased enhancement and contrast-to-noise in the arterial phase, a decrease in tumor-liver contrast-to-noise is observed during portal-venous phase, probably because of tumor perfusion and delayed washout. Tumor-liver contrast-to-noise slightly increased at 45 minutes following contrast injection, but was still lower than on precontrast images. The enhancement pattern of liver hemangiomas during serial contrast-enhanced images was similar to conventional extracellular agents. The phase 3 trials revealed improved classification and characterization of focal liver lesions by Gd-EOB-DTPA.

The per patient sensitivity for characterization was significantly higher on postcontrast images alone. It has also been demonstrated that benign hepatocyte-containing solid liver tumors, such as liver adenoma or FNH, exhibit prolonged tumor enhancement because of specific intracellular uptake of Gd-EOB-DTPA [10].

One prospective, open-label, within-patient comparison phase 3 study also contained comparative data with biphasic (arterial and portal-venous phase) helical CT [40]. The lesions detected by Gd-EOB-DTPA–enhanced MR imaging and CT were matched with histopathology. The frequency of correctly detected lesions by Gd-EOB-DTPA–enhanced MR imaging was 87.4% compared with 77.1% for CT (lesion-based analysis), and the on-site review showed that Gd-EOB-DTPA–enhanced MR imaging was superior in the detection of lesions with a diameter below 1 cm. Classification of detected lesions (benign versus malignant) was also superior for Gd-EOBDTPA–enhanced MR imaging (82.1%) compared with CT (71%). The detection rate of Gd-EOB-DTPA–enhanced MR imaging was comparable with CT but with a higher rate of detecting small lesions, and a distinctly lower rate of false-positive results. Additional information for differential diagnosis was achieved using Gd-EOB-DTPA–enhanced dynamic and static MR imaging for the characterization of malignant versus benign liver lesions and classification according to lesion type. An appropriate dose of Gd-EOB-DTPA must be used to take advantage of its high T1 relaxivity and to achieve effective perfusion enhancement. Hepatobiliary enhancement commencing at 20 minutes is an attractive feature. Gd-EOB-DTPA–enhanced MR imaging was superior to CT in the overall analysis for the pretherapeutic approach in liver imaging regarding lesion detection, localization, delineation, classification, and characterization.

Reticuloendothelial system–selective contrast agents

Reticuloendothelial system–specific contrast agents contain iron oxide particles that are selectively taken up by Kupffer cells in the liver, spleen, and bone marrow. Iron oxide particles have been developed in two different sizes. Superparamagnetic iron oxides (SPIO) have a mean iron oxide particulate size of 50 nm, whereas ultrasmall SPIO have a mean size of less than 50 nm.

Iron oxide formulations that are currently available are SPIO ferumoxides and carboxydextran-coated SPIO particles. Reticuloendothelial system–specific contrast agents are superparamagnetic causing shortening of both T2 and T1 relaxivity. T1- and T2*-weighted gradient echo and T2-weighted echo train spin echo imaging sequences are used for image acquisition. Ferumoxides are administered by intravenous infusion. One standard techniques is as follows: 15 μmol/kg SPIO concentrate is mixed in 100 mL of 5% dextrose solution and administered in drip infusion over 30 minutes [1,39]. Before the infusion the patient undergoes a noncontrast MR imaging of the liver with the use of T1-weighted gradient echo and T2-weighted sequences. Approximately 30 minutes following completion of contrast administration, the patient undergoes a repeat MR imaging with the same imaging sequences. The particles are cleared from the plasma by the reticuloendothelial system of the liver (80%) and the spleen (12%). Minimal uptake occurs in the lymph nodes and bone marrow. Ferucarbotran is administered by direct bolus injection of a small volume (<2 mL) of contrast. Serial contrast-enhanced liver imaging is performed with the use of T1-weighted gradient echo images [1,39,40]. During arterial and portal-venous phases there is no uptake in the Kupffer cells; increased signal in the vascular space and in the liver parenchyma is observed because of the presence of ferucarbotran in the liver sinusoids. In the late venous phase (90 seconds) there is increased intravascular signal and low signal in the liver parenchyma because of minimal uptake in the Kupffer cells and the intravascular blood pool effect of the agent. During the late-phase imaging (10 minutes after injection),

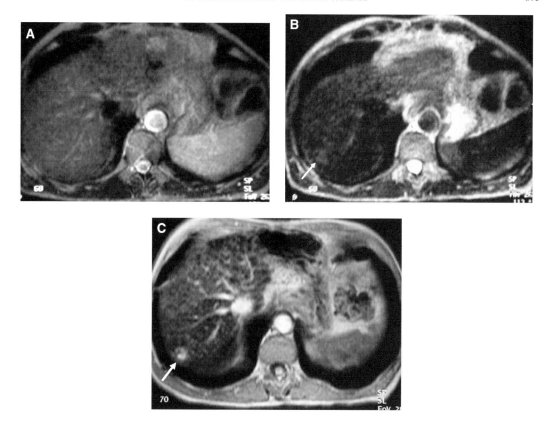

Fig. 6. A 49-year-old patient with suspect HCC. (*A*) T2-weighted fast spin echo image reveals no focal liver lesion. (*B*) After SPIO application, on T2-weighted fast spin echo image, a focal liver lesion in the posterior segment of the right liver lobe is demonstrated (*arrow*). (*C*) The same lesion is better delineated on T2*-weighted gradient echo image after SPIO application (*arrow*).

there is increased uptake of the iron particles in the Kupffer cells and liver parenchyma is rendered hypointense on both T1- and T2-weighted images. Focal liver lesions with negligible Kupffer cell content reveal higher signal relative to the contrast-mediated lower signal of the liver parenchyma (Fig. 6). FNH, hepatocellular adenomas, regenerating nodules, and dysplastic nodules contain Kupffer cells to a varying degree; their relative signal loss may parallel the signal loss in normal hepatic parenchyma after iron oxide administration [1,39–43]. Hemangiomas reveal prolonged pooling of iron oxide in the enlarged venous channels causing mild increased signal on T1-weighted images because of the blood pool effect of the agent. Comparative studies have revealed superior lesion detection rate with iron oxide–enhanced MR imaging over spiral CT. Serial gadolinium-enhanced images seem to be a better approach than the use of iron oxide–enhanced images for the detection of hepatocellular lesions, such as HCC and FNH. Limitations of SPIO-enhanced MR

imaging are relatively increased signal of cross-sectioned vessels in the low signal background liver parenchyma, and well-differentiated HCC may contain Kupffer cells and reveal contrast uptake. In patients with cirrhosis, heterogenous and diminished uptake of iron oxide by fibrotic tissue can mimic HCC [1,39].

Ultrasmall particle iron oxides are also taken up by Kupffer cells and may remain for 24 hours in the intravascular space. This blood-pool effect reveals increased vessel signal on T1-weighted images and can be used for MR angiography and for liver lesion detection and characterization [1].

Summary

This article reviews the pharmacologic and imaging features of contrast agents that are used for hepatic MR imaging. The extracellular contrast agents Gd-chelates are routinely used, and possess adequate diagnostic efficacy in the detection and characterization of most focal liver lesions because of the characteristic enhancement features of various lesions on dynamic perfusion phase imaging. The reticuloendothelial system–specific and hepatocyte-selective contrast agents have functional characterization capability because of their tissue specificity. The tissue specificity results from the affinity of the agents to normal hepatic tissue (ie, Kupffer cells or hepatocytes). The pharmacokinetic mechanisms providing this affinity, however, have limited specificity because malignant hepatocytes may still take up hepatocyte-specific contrast agents because of their functioning anion transport system, and malignant hepatocellular tumors may contain Kupffer cells. The ideal contrast agent should target tumor cells, which has not yet been developed in MR imaging.

In clinical practice, the indications and the correct choice of contrast agent for hepatic imaging depend on the clinical situation. There are three main clinical situations that require contrast-enhanced MR imaging of the liver with echocontrast cystosonography (ECS) or liver-specific contrast agents.

1. Incidental finding of a focal liver lesion in an otherwise healthy patient. In this group of patients the most common findings include hemangioma, FNH, or hepatocellular adenoma. In this group of patients, the lesions initially are depicted by ultrasound or CT, and MR imaging of the liver is required in inadequate cases. The hemangiomas are diagnosed with the use of ECS agents because of their characteristic vascular hemodynamics. The hepatocellular adenoma and the FNH are hypervascular lesions; the use of ECS agents only may not distinguish these lesions from hypervascular malignant lesions. Gd-based, hepatocyte-specific compounds are more effective in determining the nature of these lesions, even distinguishing FNH from adenomas because of their bile duct content.
2. Staging for hepatic metastases in a patient with suspect of or known extrahepatic malignancy. In this situation, ECS contrast agents may be adequate for the detection and characterization of focal liver lesions. Liver-specific contrast agents (both hepatocellular and reticuloendothelial system–specific) have been shown to increase the lesion-liver contrast and improved characterization of the detected lesions in inadequate cases.
3. Staging for HCC in a patient with liver cirrhosis or hepatitis. From a histopathologic point of view, this seems to be the most difficult task. In many cases, it is challenging for the pathologist to differentiate hyperplastic regenerative nodules from borderline HCC. In the same tumor, benign and malignant components may coexist. Differences of physiologic and functional status of the normal and malignant hepatic tissue can determine the degree of malignancy, which corresponds to the presence of functioning hepatocytes and Kupffer cells and the level of vascularization. Demonstrating the level of vascularization and lack of normal liver tissue are diagnostic determinants. The level of vascularization corresponds to the degree of contrast enhancement with ECS agents. The level of uptake of reticuloendothelial system–specific contrast agents determines the presence of functioning hepatocytes. Membrane transporter mechanism seems to be preserved in hepatocytes even if they undergo malignant transformation; hepatocyte-specific contrast agents are taken up by the preserved membrane transport system. The hepatocyte-selective contrast agents seem not to add substantial diagnostic information on vascularization during the distribution phase. Combined use of ferumoxides and Gd-chelate–enhanced MR imaging is reported to increase the diagnostic efficacy of MR imaging for the evaluation of HCC. Nevertheless, this approach is very costly.

References

[1] Semelka RC, Helmberger TK. Contrast agents for MR imaging of the liver. Radiology 2001;218:27–38.
[2] Cavagna FM, Dapra M, Castelli PM, et al. Trends and developments in MRI contrast agent research. Eur Radiol 1997;7(Suppl 5):222–4.
[3] Earls JP, Rofsky NM, DeCorato DR, et al. Hepatic arterial-phase dynamic enhanced MR imaging: optimization with a test examination and a power injector. Radiology 1997;202:268–73.
[4] Webb JA, Thomsen HS, Morcos SK. The use of iodinated and gadolinium contrast media during pregnancy and lactation. Eur Radiol 2005;15(6):1234–40.
[5] Semelka RC, Worawattankul S, Kelekis NL, et al. Liver lesion detection, characterization, and effect on patient management: comparison of single phase spiral CT and current MR techniques. J Magn Reson Imaging 1997;7:1040–7.
[6] Semelka RC, Martin DR, Balci NC, et al. Focal liver lesions: comparison of dual-phase CT and multisequence multiplanar MR imaging including dynamic

gadolinium enhancement. J Magn Reson Imaging 2001;13:397–401.

[7] Whitney WS, Herfkens RJ, Jeffrey RB, et al. Dynamic breath-hold multiplanar spoiled gradient-recalled MR imaging with gadolinium enhancement for differentiating hemangiomas from malignancies at 1.5 T. Radiology 1993;189:863–70.

[8] Hamm B, Mahfouz AE, Taupitz M, et al. Liver metastases: improved detection with dynamic gadolinium-enhanced MR imaging? Radiology 1997;202:677–82.

[9] Reimer P, Saini S, Kwong KK, et al. Dynamic gadolinium-enhanced echo-planar MR imaging of the liver: effect of pulse sequence and dose on enhancement. J Magn Reson Imaging 1994;4:331–5.

[10] Reimer P, Schneider G, Schima W. Hepatobiliary contrast agents for contrast-enhanced MRI of the liver: properties, clinical development and applications. Eur Radiol 2004;14:559–78.

[11] Wang C. Mangafodipir trisodium (MnDPDP)-enhanced magnetic resonance imaging of the liver and pancreas. Acta Radiol Suppl 1998;415:1–31.

[12] Wang C, Ahlstrom H, Ekholm S. Diagnostic efficacy of MnDPDP in MR imaging of the liver: a phase III multicentre study. Acta Radiol 1997;38:643–9.

[13] Aicher KP, Laniado M, Kopp AF, et al. Mn-DPDP-enhanced MR imaging of malignant liver lesions: efficacy and safety in 20 patients. J Magn Reson Imaging 1993;3:731–7.

[14] Bartolozzi C, Donati F, Cioni D, et al. MnDPDP-enhanced MRI vs dual-phase spiral CT in the detection of hepatocellular carcinoma in cirrhosis. Eur Radiol 2000;10:1697–702.

[15] Marti-Bonmati L, Fog AF, de Beeck BO, et al. Safety and efficacy of mangafodipir trisodium in patients with liver lesions and cirrhosis. Eur Radiol 2003;13:1685–92.

[16] de Haen C, Lorusso V, Luzzani F, et al. Hepatic transport of gadobenate dimeglumine in TR-rats. Acad Radiol 1996;3:S452–4.

[17] Kirchin MA, Pirovano G, Venetianer C, et al. Gadobenate dimeglumine (Gd-BOPTA), an overview. Invest Radiol 1998;33:798–809.

[18] Spinazzi A, Lorusso V, Pirovano G, et al. Safety, tolerance, biodistribution, and MR imaging enhancement of the liver with gadobenate dimeglumine: results of clinical pharmacologic and pilot imaging studies in nonpatient and patient volunteers. Acad Radiol 1999;6:282–91.

[19] de Haen C, Gozzini L. Solubletype hepatobiliary contrast agents for MR imaging. J Magn Reson Imaging 1993;3:179–86.

[20] Schima W, Petersein J, Hahn PF, et al. Contrast enhanced MR imaging of the liver: comparison between Gd-BOPTA and Mangafodipir. J Magn Reson Imaging 1997;7:130–5.

[21] de Haen C, La Ferla R, Maggioni F. Gadobenate dimeglumine 0.5 M solution for injection (Multi-Hance) as contrast agent for magnetic resonance imaging of the liver: mechanistic studies in animals. J Comput Assist Tomogr 1999;23:S169–79.

[22] Cavagna FM, Maggioni F, Castelli PM, et al. Gadolinium chelates with weak binding to serum proteins: a new class of high-efficiency, general purpose contrast agents for magnetic resonance imaging. Invest Radiol 1997;32:780–96.

[23] Schuhmann-Giampieri G. Liver contrast media for magnetic resonance imaging: interrelations between pharmacokinetics and imaging. Invest Radiol 1993;28:753–61.

[24] Spinazzi A, Lorusso V, Pirovano G, et al. Multihance clinical pharmacology: biodistribution and MR enhancement of the liver. Acad Radiol 1998;5(Suppl 1):S86–9 [discussion: S93-4].

[25] Powers C, Ros PR, Stoupis C, et al. Primary liver neoplasms: MR imaging with pathologic correlation. Radiographics 1994;14:459–82.

[26] Mahfouz AE, Hamm B, Wolf KJ. Peripheral washout: a sign of malignancy on dynamic gadolinium enhanced MR images of focal liver lesions. Radiology 1994;190:49–52.

[27] Semelka RC, Brown ED, Ascher SM, et al. Hepatic hemangiomas: a multi-institutional study of appearance on T2-weighted and serial gadolinium-enhanced gradient-echo MR images. Radiology 1994;192:401–6.

[28] Hamm B, Thoeni RF, Gould RG, et al. Focal liver lesions: characterization with nonenhanced and dynamic contrast material enhanced MR imaging. Radiology 1994;190:417–23.

[29] Hamm B, Mahfouz AE, Taupitz M, et al. Liver metastases: improved detection with dynamic gadolinium-enhanced MR imaging? Radiology 1997;202:677–82.

[30] Kuwatsuru R, Kadoya M, Ohtomo K, et al. Comparison of gadobenate dimeglumine with gadopentetate dimeglumine for magnetic resonance imaging of liver tumors. Invest Radiol 2001;36:632–41.

[31] Petersein J, Spinazzi A, Giovagnoni A, et al. Focal liver lesions: evaluation of the efficacy of gadobenate dimeglumine in MR imaging: a multicenter phase III clinical study. Radiology 2000;215:727–36.

[32] Schneider G, Maas R, Schultze Kool L, et al. Low-dose gadobenate dimeglumine versus standard dose gadopentetate dimeglumine for contrast-enhanced magnetic resonance imaging of the liver: an intra-individual crossover comparison. Invest Radiol 2003;38:85–94.

[33] Morana G, Grazioli L, Schneider G, et al. Hyper-vascular hepatic lesions: dynamic and late enhancement pattern with Gd-BOPTA. Acad Radiol 2002;9(Suppl 2):476–9.

[34] Grazioli L, Morana G, Kirchin MA, et al. MRI of focal nodular hyperplasia (FNH) with gadobenate dimeglumine (Gd-BOPTA) and SPIO (ferumoxides): an intra-individual comparison. J Magn Reson Imaging 2003;17:593–602.

[35] Weinmann HJ, Schuhmann-Giampieri G, Schmitt-Willich H, et al. A new lipophilic gadolinium chelate

as a tissue-specific contrast medium for MRI. Magn Reson Med 1991;22:233–7.

[36] Schuhmann-Giampieri G, Schmitt-Willich H, Press WR, et al. Preclinical evaluation of Gd-EOBDTPA as a contrast agent in MR imaging of the hepatobiliary system. Radiology 1992;183:59–64.

[37] Hamm B, Staks T, Muhler A. Phase I clinical evaluation of Gd-EOB-DTPA as a hepatobiliary MR contrast agent: safety, pharmacokinetics, and MR imaging. Radiology 1995;195:785–92.

[38] Reimer P, Rummeny EJ, Shamsi K, et al. Phase II clinical evaluation of Gd-EOB-DTPA: dose, safety aspects, and pulse sequence. Radiology 1996;199: 177–83.

[39] Shamsi K. Gd-EOB-DTPA (Eovist), a liver specific contrast agent for MRI: results of a placebo controlled, double blind dose ranging study in patients with focal liver lesions. Presented at the Tenth scientific meeting and exhibition of the International Society for Magnetic Resonance in Medicine. Honolulu, Hawaii, May 18–24, 2002.

[40] Huppertz A, Balzer T, Blakeborough A, et al. Improved detection of focal liver lesions in MRI: a multicenter comparison of Gd-EOB-DTPA with intraoperative findings. Radiology 2004;230:266–75.

[41] Bellin MF, Zaim S, Auberton E, et al. Liver metastases: safety and efficacy of detection with superparamagnetic iron oxide in MR imaging. Radiology 1994; 193:657–63.

[42] Winter III TC, Freeny PC, Nghiem HV, et al. MR imaging with i.v. superparamagnetic iron oxide: efficacy in the detection of focal hepatic lesions. AJR Am J Roentgenol 1993;161:1191–8.

[43] Weissleder R, Elizondo G, Wittenberg J, et al. Ultrasmall superparamagnetic iron oxide: characterization of a new class of contrast agents for MR imaging. Radiology 1990;175:489–93.

Radiol Clin N Am 43 (2005) 899–914

RADIOLOGIC
CLINICS
of North America

Local Therapeutic Treatments for Focal Liver Disease

Susan M. Weeks, MD*, Charles Burke, MD

Department of Radiology, School of Medicine, University of North Carolina at Chapel Hill, 2016 Old Clinic Building, Campus Box 7510, Chapel Hill, NC 27599–7510, USA

Patients diagnosed with primary hepatic malignancies or metastases to the liver remain a difficult population to treat. A small percentage of these people can undergo surgical resection or transplantation. The remaining nonsurgical aggregate does not often benefit from conventional radiation and chemotherapy; minimally invasive means either to cure or palliate these patients are a requirement for complete cancer care. This article discusses image-guided local therapies used to treat this difficult patient population, focusing predominantly on radiofrequency ablation (RFA).

Tumors

Hepatocellular carcinoma

Hepatocellular carcinoma (HCC) is the third leading cause of cancer-related deaths worldwide, responsible for approximately 1,000,000 deaths yearly. Within the United States, there has been an 80% increase in the annual incidence of HCC over the last 15 to 20 years, likely caused by the marked increase in hepatitis C. HCC carries with it a dismal prognosis. If left untreated, median life expectancy is 6 to 9 months with mortality approaching 100% at 5 years [1,2]. Conventional chemotherapy and radiation have little proved benefit for these patients, and surgical resection or transplantation offer the best hope for survival. Only 13% to 35% of patients with

HCC are candidates for resection, however, with surgical contraindications including multifocal disease, tumor location precluding successful negative margins, insufficient hepatic reserve, and comorbidities precluding surgery [3,4]. Overall, survival rates after partial hepatectomy for HCC range from 35% to 50% at 5 years, with an operative mortality of 5% to 10% [5].

Although resection removes the offending lesion, it does not cure the underlying disease process that may lead to recurrence. Approximately 50% of patients with HCC who undergo surgical resection develop new lesions within 2 years, and as many as 70% have a recurrence within 5 years [5,6]. For this reason, liver transplantation can be advantageous in this patient population. Although mortality rates following transplantation are only slightly increased with respect to resection, the survival rates for liver transplantation are better, with 5-year survival rates reported at 63% to 74%.

Not all patients with HCC are candidates for transplantation. Because of the finite number of organs available, the United Network for Organ Sharing has developed a scoring system based on the Model for End-Stage Liver Disease criteria to establish priority for organ recipients [1,7]. Under this system, transplantation can be considered in patients with a single HCC smaller than 5 cm or no more than three hepatomas 3 cm or less. Given these strict size criteria, techniques to control tumor growth while awaiting transplantation take on great importance.

Hepatic metastases

Colorectal carcinoma is the second leading cause of cancer-related deaths in the United States. Approxi-

---

* Corresponding author.
E-mail address: sue_weeks@med.unc.edu
(S.M. Weeks).

radiologic.theclinics.com

mately 15% to 25% of patients with colon cancer have liver metastases at the time of presentation; an additional 20% develop hepatic metastases during the course of their disease [8]. This becomes critically important because patient mortality is most commonly caused by metastatic disease, with a median survival of 5 to 10 months and a 5-year survival of 2% to 8% if no treatment is initiated [9–11]. Eradication of hepatic metastases is essential for long-term survival. Because only 5% to 20% of patients with hepatic metastatic disease are considered candidates for surgical resection, however, there is a terrific need for local, reliable, alternative methods to treat local hepatic disease in the nonsurgical candidate [12].

Thermal ablation

Thermal ablative techniques destroy tumor and a rim of normal tissue around the tumor (similar to a surgical resection margin), while maintaining the normal surrounding parenchyma. When heat is applied to cells, they go through predictable reactions, with the degree of tissue damage being dependent on the level and duration of heating [13]. When a heat source is applied to tissue, at 45°C cells become edematous and microvascular flow changes occur [14]. If this heat is applied for several hours, cell death may result. At 50 to 55°C irreversible cell changes occur in as little as 4 to 6 minutes with effaced sinusoids and stasis of flow evident microscopically. Immediate tissue coagulation occurs at temperatures between 60 and 100°C, with vaporization occurring at temperatures above 100°C. Ideally, thermal ablation should homogeneously heat the target tissue to 60 to 100°C. When temperature elevation is inadequate, incomplete tumor destruction may occur, leaving residual disease. At temperatures over 100°C, vaporization results in a barrier to further tissue heating and impedes dispersion of heat and restricts total heat deposition [13].

Radiofrequency ablation

Although there are many sources available to apply heat to tumor (high-frequency ultrasound, laser, microwave), RFA has gained the most popularity in the United States. RFA was first described as a local treatment for hepatic malignancies in two separate reports published in 1990 [15,16]. An insulated needle electrode is placed into a tumor, usually with imaging guidance, and then attached to a generator. Grounding pads are placed on the patient to create a

closed circuit. Power is delivered from the generator to the active tip of the electrode, resulting in high-frequency current (200–1200 kHz) deposition within the target tissue [13]. The oscillating current agitates the ions within the tissue around the needle electrode, generating friction and heat. Heat is greatest at the tip of the electrode, because this is the area of strongest electrical field. Ideally, this heat is dispersed homogeneously from the electrode throughout the tissue being treated, while minimizing char and vaporization, which impede heat deposition and dispersion. This is best described by the bioheat equation described by Pennes in 1948 [17,18]: coagulation necrosis = energy deposited × local tissue interactions – heat loss.

Forty two years later, McGahan and coworkers [15] determined that a single monopolar electrode could reliably create a 1.6-cm diameter region of coagulative necrosis. This small treatment size was not applicable in and of itself to the everyday treatment of malignant tumors. In line with the bioheat equation listed previously, modifications of this initial probe design from 1990 have been created to make this technology clinically useful.

Multitined expandable probes

Expandable, multitined needle electrodes were developed to increase burn diameter and homogeneity. Multiple tines allow the deposition of heat at multiple locations within a tumor. These focal areas of heating then coalesce to form a larger, homogeneously treated burn diameter. By using such technology, LeVeen [19] demonstrated reproducible burns of up to 3.5 cm in an in vivo porcine liver, a marked improvement over the 1.6 cm burn seen with a single monopolar needle electrode. Improvements in this tine technology, including an increase in generator power, and changes in the geometry of the tine configuration have led to coagulation diameters approaching 6 cm [20]. Additionally, the simultaneous instillation of saline solution during RFA has demonstrated burn diameters approaching 7 cm, discussed later in this article.

The RITA (Mountain View, California) and Radiotherapeutics (Sunnyvale, California) systems take advantage of this multitined technology. The nonsaline-infused RITA needle electrode systems consist of an insulated needle and nine deployable, curved tines. The diameter of the ablation zone is dependent on the diameter to which the tines are deployed. When fully deployed, the device tines have a diameter up to 5 cm. A 250-W generator supplies an alternating current operating at 460 kHz. Five of the tines have temperature sensors that are used to monitor the ablation procedure. Tines are progressively deployed from 2 cm to the target diameter (3–5 cm) when target temperature is achieved at each level. A flexible probe is also available, which facilitates usage in CT scanners where space in the gantry may be limited [21].

The Radiotherapeutics electrode needle is 14 gauge and comes either insulated or as part of a coaxial system. The coaxial system includes an insulated introducer sheath and stylet. The electrodes are connected to a 480-kHz generator that is capable of generating up to 200 W of power. The Radiotherapeutics system monitors the ablation progress by measuring tissue impedance. Tissue impedance is a function of resistance and rises as tissues begin to coagulate. Needle electrodes are available up to 5 cm in diameter.

Internally cooled electrodes

To decrease char and vaporization at the electrode tip, internally cooled electrodes were developed. Remembering the bioheat equation, a decrease in vaporization should result in an increase in heat deposition and an increase in coagulative necrosis. The Radionics Cool-tip RFA system (Tyco, Burlington, Massachusetts) consists of either a single 17-gauge electrode or a cluster of three electrodes connected to a 480-kHz generator that generates up to 250 W of power [22]. The clustered electrodes are spaced 0.5 mm apart and are internally cooled by chilled saline, which is continuously circulated through the electrodes and then drained externally. This cooling results in cooling of the tissue adjacent to the electrode tip, minimizing local impedance during delivery of current. The device measures this impedance and adjusts the power output accordingly to increase overall ablation volume. Treatments are typically completed within 12 to 15 minutes, and burn diameters are reported to approach 5 cm [23,24].

Perfusion electrodes

Perfusion electrodes allow the instillation of saline into the tissue to be ablated while ablation occurs, in hopes of increasing the volume treated. This has been demonstrated in experimental settings to be effective using both normal saline and hypertonic saline [25,26]. The mechanism behind this is complex, but may include increasing the area of the active surface electrode, reducing tissue vaporization, or improving thermal conduction [27]. RITA has created a 7-cm needle electrode that infuses saline solution into the

surrounding tissues by the deployed tines during the ablation. A second system, by Berchtold (Tuttlingen, Germany), consists of a single 14-gauge electrode needle that is connected to a 375-kHz generator capable of generating 60 W of power [22,24]. The monopolar electrode infuses saline solution through side holes at the tip of the needle during the ablation procedure. Ablations are performed by delivering 50 W of power for three separate 5-minute intervals.

Local tissue interactions

To increase consistent burn diameters with RFA, improving local tissue interactions by improving heat conduction and altering thermal and electrical conductivity of treated tissues has been investigated [27]. Perfusion electrodes described previously are based on this concept. The instillation of fluid into the tumor before or during RFA results in heating of that liquid, which results in dispersion of the heated liquid and resultant increase in thermal energy deposition. The mechanism of action, however, is likely quite complex and multifactorial. Goldberg and coworkers [25] investigated the effects of concentration and volume on coagulative volume, and found that increased saline concentrations caused an increase in electrical conductivity and enabled increased energy deposition into tissue, but that this did not hold true at markedly increased levels of tissue conductivity. Other effects on local tissue interactions are described in the combined therapies section.

Heat loss

Clinical RFA results have not followed advances seen in ex vivo experiments with respect to result reproducibility and increase in burn diameter. This is likely because of the local tissue environment, including adjacent structures, both vascular and otherwise. Convincing in vivo pig data from Lu and coworkers [28] clearly demonstrated the "heat sink" effect in the presence of vessels greater than 3 mm in diameter. These same authors investigated the effect of vessels 3 mm and greater on clinical tumor recurrence rates, and found that a peritumoral vessel at least 3 mm in diameter was a strong independent predictor of incomplete tumor destruction after RFA [29]. It makes sense, then, that improved RFA strategies include methods to control neighboring vascularity during ablation. Experiments using both pharmacologic and mechanical control of vascularity in proximity to treatment regions have been performed both in the laboratory and in clinical settings. Using an in vivo porcine model, Goldberg and coworkers [30] looked at the effects of intra-arterial halothane and vasopressin injection on burn diameter, and found excellent correlation between diminished blood flow and increasing coagulation diameter. Mechanical control, including vascular embolization, temporary balloon occlusion, and the Pringle maneuver, has been studied (Fig. 1). In an in vivo porcine model, Patterson and coworkers [31] found that by using the Pringle maneuver, they could successfully increase overall burn volume from 6.5 to 35 cm^3. Rossi and coworkers [32] modulated hepatic arterial blood flow in 62 patients during RFA, and found they could obtain on average a 4.7-cm burn using a 3-cm RITA probe. Yamakado and coworkers [33] per-

formed the Pringle maneuver in a subset of patients with colorectal metastases undergoing RFA and demonstrated an increase in coagulation diameter from 2.5 to 4 cm.

Combined therapies

Without reviewing clinical studies, it should be clear that the current RFA technology can reliably treat a 3-cm lesion with one needle placement, providing a 1-cm margin around the circumference of the tumor. Many patients with hepatic tumoral involvement have tumors larger than 3 cm, however, and no good treatment option available to them. In

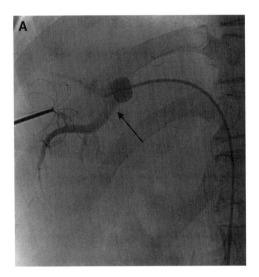
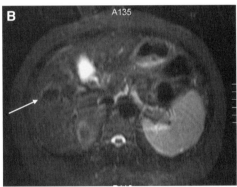
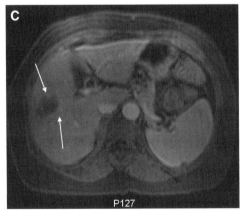

Fig. 1. (*A*) Static fluoroscopic image obtained during RFA of an HCC abutting a large branch of the right hepatic vein (*arrow*). An occlusion balloon has been placed by a femoral vein approach to improve the therapeutic burn at the tumor margin abutting the vein. (*B*) Short tau inversion recovery sequence after RFA demonstrates dark signal in the tumor bed (*arrow*). (*C*) Contrast-enhanced three-dimensional volume interpolated body examination demonstrates no enhancement within the treatment bed suggestive of residual tumor. Note the hepatic vein abutting the treatment site (*arrows*).

addition to blood flow modulation, combined therapies have been and are being developed to increase volume of coagulative necrosis created by the current RFA technology, in hopes of expanding the use of this modality. RFA in concert with direct tumoral injection, chemical ablation, chemoembolization, embolization, and chemotherapy have been and are being studied both in the laboratory and clinically.

Percutaneous ethanol injection is an effective treatment for small hepatomas. Lee and coworkers [34], when combining this treatment with RFA in an in vivo rabbit liver, found significantly longer coagulation diameters when compared with treatment groups undergoing either conventional RFA or percutaneous ethanol injection alone. The authors also demonstrated increased treatment zone irregularity, however, when compared with conventional RFA [34]. Kurokohchi and coworkers [35,36] compared RFA following bolus injection of ethanol with standard RFA in 73 patients with HCC and found significant increases in coagulation necrosis in those patients undergoing combined therapy. These same authors investigated the effect of RFA with percutaneous ethanol injection in patients with lesions located in regions that are classically difficult to treat, including those abutting major vascular structures. They found complete necrosis of these tumors without an associated increase in complication rate [36].

Similarly, Lee and coworkers [34] evaluated the effect of percutaneous acetic acid injection in conjunction with RFA in an in vivo rabbit model, comparing this treatment strategy with RFA and percutaneous acetic acid injection alone. They found a significant increase in burn diameter with the combined treatment, and although there were an increased number of complications in that study group compared with the group undergoing standard RFA, the number did not reach significance. In the past, both of these treatment responses have been attributed to the toxic effects of both percutaneous ethanol injection and percutaneous acetic acid injection. Ahmed and coworkers [37], however, investigated the effect of percutaneous acetic acid injection alone and in combination with RFA, using a hypovascular canine tumor model. In this study, they evaluated the effect of differing acetic acid concentrations diluted in both distilled water and saturated sodium chloride solution. Controls included standard RFA, 36% sodium chloride injection with and without RFA, and distilled water injection. They found an increase in coagulation with increasing acetic acid concentrations, and increased coagulation with combination RFA and percutaneous acetic acid injection

compared with either treatment alone. They found maximum heating and coagulation when 10% AA was diluted in sodium chloride, however, with greater radiofrequency heating when tumors were pretreated with acetic acid in sodium chloride rather than diluted in water. They conclude from this study that, in the model used, increased tumor ablation was more likely caused by significant alterations in electrical conductivity rather than the inherent ablative effects of acetic acid.

RFA in conjunction with transcatheter arterial chemoembolization and transcatheter arterial embolization has been investigated. A recent paper by Yamakado and coworkers [33] evaluated the combined effects of RFA following transcatheter arterial chemoembolization in 64 patients with 108 lesions. A total of 65 lesions were ≤ 3 cm, 32 were between 3 and 5 cm, and 11 were between 5.1 and 12 cm. Seventy-four were nodular and 34 were either multinodular or infiltrative. Using imaging criteria to determine tumor necrosis, they found complete necrosis in all lesions, with no recurrences in the first two study groups regardless of tumor morphology, during a mean follow-up of 12.5 months. In the large tumor group, two of six nonnodular recurrences were identified beyond the thermal lesions initially created. The authors concluded that transcatheter arterial chemoembolization in combination with RFA was effective in treating small and intermediate-sized hepatomas, and may be successful in treating large hepatomas. They noted that treatment of nonnodular lesions remains difficult.

The use of chemotherapy in conjunction with RFA has been studied both in the laboratory and the clinical setting. Goldberg and coworkers [38] treated rat mammary adenocarcinomas with intratumoral injection of doxorubicin followed by RFA, and found significantly increased coagulation diameters than when compared with either treatment alone. Specifically, the authors found the greatest effect when the doxorubicin was administered 30 minutes following RFA, and postulated that the cells located at the periphery of the burn may have suffered sublethal injury that predisposed them to death once hit with the second insult (RFA). Goldberg and coworkers [39] subsequently investigated the effect of intravenous liposomal doxorubicin injection and RFA in five patients with seven tumors, comparing them with five patients undergoing RFA. In this randomized study, using multiphasic CT, the authors found no difference in amount of tumor destruction immediately following RFA. Two to 4 weeks after treatment, however, the group undergoing combination therapy had an increase in tumor destruction, up to 15 mm in diameter. This resulted in a median volumetric increase in tissue kill of 32%. Additionally, tumor destruction was more complete and notable in areas of difficult treatment, including perivascular regions. This was in stark contrast to scans obtained in patients undergoing routine RFA, where a decrease in volume was identified on concurrent follow-up scans.

Clinical considerations

Patient selection

When evaluating a potential patient for RFA, the ideal candidate has three or fewer small (less than 3 cm) lesions, all surrounded by hepatic parenchyma. Lesions should be more than 1 cm away from any large vessel or adjacent organ. Because there are very few perfect patients, the goal of therapy needs to be discussed with the patient during initial consultation to ensure that there are no unrealistic expectations, and that all involved parties are acting on the same premise. During this initial consultation, imaging is reviewed; pertinent history is obtained; laboratory values are acquired and reviewed as needed (liver function tests, alpha fetoprotein, platelets, prothrombin time, and partial thromboplastin time); risks and benefits are discussed; and consent is signed.

Review of the cross-sectional imaging remains an important part of the consultation. Although the authors prefer contrast-enhanced MR imaging, which has been shown to be more sensitive than multiple-phase CT for the detection of focal hepatic lesions, biphasic or triphasic CT scan is generally more widely available [40–42]. The cross-sectional imaging study quantifies lesion number, size, morphologic subtype, and location. Larger lesions are more difficult completely to necrose. Livraghi and coworkers [43] cited rates of complete necrosis for small (lesions ≤ 3 cm) HCC of 90%. In lesions 3.1 to 5 cm and greater than 5 cm, the rate of complete necrosis following RFA dropped to 71% and 24%, respectively [44]. In a study evaluating RFA in the transplant population, the complete response rate for lesions larger than 3 cm was only 29% [45]. Additionally, as lesion size increases, tumoral sub-

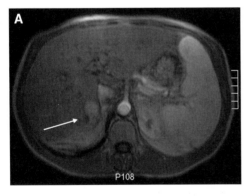
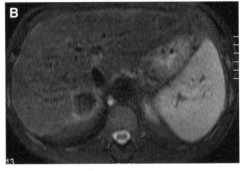
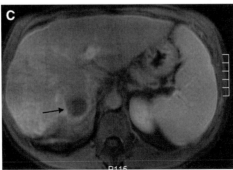

Fig. 2. (*A*) Postcontrasted fast low angle shot (FLASH) image demonstrates an enhancing HCC involving the subcapsular portion of the liver (*arrow*). (*B*) Follow-up MR image 1 month later demonstrates dark T2 signal at the tumor bed. (*C*) Postenhanced FLASH images demonstrate a thin rim of enhancement corresponding with inflammation at this site (*arrow*). The burn site is larger now than the original lesion.

type increases in importance. Larger, infiltrative lesions are more difficult to treat than smaller, well-circumscribed lesions, using a variety of treatment modalities including RFA [33].

Almost as important as size is lesion location [13,45,46]. Tumors demonstrating a higher recurrence risk include surface lesions and perivascular lesions [2,13,46,47]. Subcapsular lesions and lesions adjacent to the diaphragm may be better approached laparoscopically, although a recent report by Poon and coworkers [48] demonstrated successful percutaneous ablation of subcapsular lesions without associated increase in morbidity or incomplete treatment (Fig. 2). Vessels larger than 3 mm are thought to result in a heat sink, making it difficult to achieve adequate temperatures for effective tissue coagulation in perivascular locations. This might be overcome by using a combination therapy, such as an infusate and RFA [37]. Evaluation of lesion location indicates potential postablation complications. Biliary system injuries, including stricture, subsequent liver failure, cholecystitis, and biloma formation, have been reported [49–52]. Injury to a structure in close proximity to the planned ablation site can be avoided by using such techniques as the instillation of saline or water or placement of a balloon between the burn site and vital organ to increase the distance between the two just before RFA.

During the patient consultation, the authors also determine which imaging modality to use for the procedure. At the authors' institution, if the lesion cannot be clearly visualized with ultrasound guidance, a noncontrasted liver CT is obtained. Occasionally, the lesion cannot be seen with either modality. In this case, an alternative approach for the patient with HCC is intra-arterial ethiodol-enhanced CT (Fig. 3). Ethiodol-enhanced CT has been shown to be sensitive for localization of small HCC and has also been used safely and effectively to target lesions [53,54]. Alternatively, as ultrasound contrast agents become widely available, more lesions may be visible with transabdominal ultrasound guidance [55]. Recently, work has been done demonstrating the feasibility of using MR imaging guidance for RFA, although this is not yet widely available [56]. If the lesion is not visible using any of these modalities, then referral for laparoscopic guidance may be necessary.

There are few contraindications to RFA of liver lesions. Patients with uncorrectable coagulopathies are at a much higher risk for significant bleeding complications, even with track ablation. Caution should be practiced in patients with prior bilioenteric anastomoses, because these patients are thought to be at higher risk for developing postablation cholangitis or hepatic abscess formation [57].

Procedure

Percutaneous RFA often can be performed on an outpatient basis. An overnight admission might be indicated in patients with poor initial hepatic function, persistent sedative effect or pain following the procedure, unexpected complication, or significant distance between home and hospital. Some authors have advocated the use of preprocedural antibiotics, although this is controversial [50,52]. The patient is placed on the procedure table and grounding pads are applied to the patient's thighs. The appropriate area is sterilely prepared and draped after lesion location is confirmed. Intravenous sedation is administered and a local anesthetic is used. Uncommonly, a patient requires general anesthesia, although this may be necessary in patients with poor hepatic function and uncontrollable pain during ablation. A needle electrode allowing a 1-cm margin is then chosen to perform the burn. If multiple burns are necessary, then this is either planned with sequential needle electrode placement, or all needle electrodes may be placed at one time and then the burn created. Needle electrode positioning should follow the recommendations specified by each manufacturer; the electrode is connected to the generator and a burn is created per the manufacturer's algorithm. The size of the ablation zone should allow for at least a 1-cm margin around the circumference of the lesion, such that a 3-cm lesion requires a 5-cm burn [13]. This should treat microscopic extension of tumor and is analogous to a 1-cm surgical margin.

For lesions measuring 3 cm or less, single probe placements often achieve an appropriate burn. Successful treatment of larger lesions, however, requires a more elaborate treatment plan. Mathematical models have been constructed demonstrating how multiple overlapping burns can be used to achieve complete lesion necrosis with an acceptable 1-cm margin. Many overlapping burns may be required, however, to ensure adequate margins on all sides. To treat a 5-cm diameter lesion with a 3-cm probe adequately, 12 to 14 overlapping spheres are required [13,58,59]. This is a major impetus for the body of work evaluating combination therapies, discussed previously.

One of the current difficulties with RFA is assessing the adequacy of treatment at the time of the procedure. When the procedure is being performed with ultrasound guidance, the area of ablation tends to become hyperechoic (Fig. 4). Small bubbles may

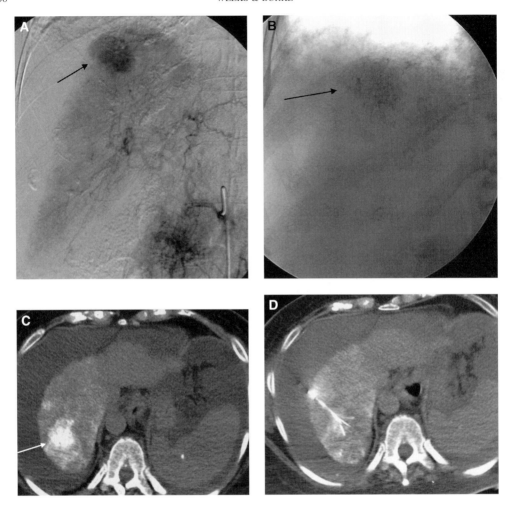

Fig. 3. Ethiodol-enhanced RFA. (*A*) Initial arteriogram demonstrating enhancing dome HCC not visible at ultrasound or with noncontrasted CT (*arrow*). (*B*) Digital image of HCC after the selective catheterization and instillation of ethiodol to the tumor (*arrow*). (*C*) Noncontrasted CT image demonstrating marked uptake of ethiodol by the tumor (*arrow*). (*D*) Using ethiodol-enhanced CT, the lesion is accessed with a RITA needle probe and RFA is completed.

even be seen within the nearby hepatic veins. This is the result of microbubble formation that occurs when the temperature within the tissues reaches 95°C [60]. It is tempting to use the size of this hyperechoic region to judge the amount of tissue ablated, and one study did find a positive correlation in the size of this hyperechoic zone and the mean diameter of tissue necrosis [60]. It should not be used as a basis for determining adequacy of treatment, however, because it can overestimate and underestimate the true area of coagulation [55,60]. There are some early data suggesting that contrast-enhanced Doppler ultrasound may be useful in immediately assessing adequacy of treatment [61]. Some authors have also advocated obtaining an immediate postprocedural contrast-

enhanced CT to evaluate for residual disease and immediate complications [62].

At the conclusion of the procedure, most devices allow for thermocoagulation of the needle track. This has two primary benefits. First, track ablation helps to reduce the risk of bleeding complications. Second, track ablation may reduce the risk of seeding the needle track. After the procedure, the patient is transferred to the recovery area, where the authors recommend monitoring for a minimum of 4 hours. Following recovery, if the patient is awake and pain is adequately controlled, the patient is discharged home and given instructions and a telephone number to call should any problems arise overnight. Patients are then called the following day to ascertain if any prob-

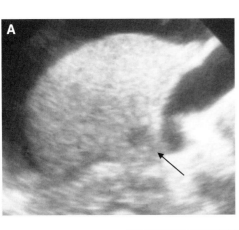
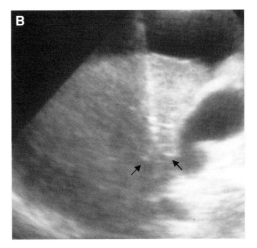
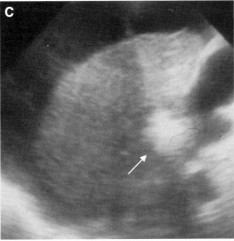

Fig. 4. Microbubble formation. (*A*) Ultrasound at time of RFA demonstrates 2-cm, hypoechoic HCC deep within the liver (*arrow*). (*B*) Tines can be clearly identified within the lesion after having been deployed (*arrows*). (*C*) Following 15 minutes of ablation time, a larger mass of microbubbles is identified at the level of the burn and obscures the initial lesion (*arrow*).

lems occurred since discharge. Return clinic appointments and repeat scanning are scheduled at 4 to 6 weeks after the initial ablation to determine adequacy of treatment and address any patient concerns.

Postablation imaging

Before embarking on a discussion of the findings on postablation imaging, it is important to review the pathologic changes occurring in the area of ablation. Microscopically, during and immediately after RFA four distinct zones are present around the radiofrequency probe [14]. Closest to the probe, there is coagulated tissue with increased endothelial leakiness, cellular edema of the hepatic sinusoids, and

infiltration of carbon microparticles [14]. With increasing distance from the probe, there is improved microvascular perfusion and normalization of cellular morphology. Grossly, three distinct zones are seen: (1) a central area of necrosis, (2) a hemorrhagic rim, and (3) an outer pink rim [63]. These zones can persist up to 5 months and represent central necrosis with outer granulation tissue. At anywhere from 2 to 12 weeks, a two-zone appearance predominates [63]. The inner zone is comprised of coagulated necrotic tissue with an outer rim of fibrous tissue and chronic inflammatory cells [64]. These distinct zones give the postablation site a distinctive appearance on follow-up imaging.

Just as with the preablation imagining, either contrast-enhanced CT or MR imaging may be used

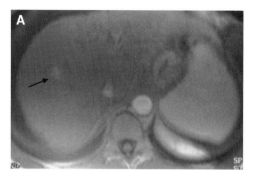 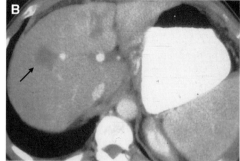

Fig. 5. (*A*) Pre-RFA contrasted MR image demonstrates a small, early enhancing mass indicative of HCC (*arrow*). (*B*) Two months following ablation, contrasted CT demonstrates a larger, hypodense, nonenhancing lesion indicative of a successful burn (*arrow*).

for postablation follow-up. MR imaging, however, may be slightly more sensitive in evaluating for residual disease [65]. There is some early work available investigating the use of contrast-enhanced ultrasound and positron emission tomography for the evaluation of residual disease and for postablation surveillance [55,61,66,67]. Some authors recommend obtaining an imaging study either immediately after the ablation or within 1 week of the ablation to evaluate for residual tumor [13,68]. Other authors recommend waiting 1 month before obtaining the first imaging study to avoid confusion between acute postablation changes and residual tumor [2,59]. Imaging is then performed at 3 and 6 months, and then at 1 year. If there is no evidence of recurrent or residual disease, the patient should then undergo routine follow-up imaging every 6 to 12 months.

When using contrast-enhanced CT for follow-up, necrotic tissue appears hypodense on all scans [69,70]. The size of the lesion may initially appear larger than the original lesion, because of the 1-cm circumferential margin obtained during RFA (Fig. 5). The lesion should not enlarge, however, during follow-up; an enlarging postablation zone is highly suggestive of recurrent tumor even in the absence of abnormal enhancement [70,71]. Within the 1 to 2 months after ablation, a thin rim of enhancement may be seen around the treated area [69,71]. This represents the zone of fibrosis and granulation tissue seen pathologically [64,69]. Loss of sharp delineation of the ablation margin, increased nodularity of the lesion, or crescentic thickening around the ablation site may all be findings indicative of residual or recurrent disease [69,70]. Particular attention should be paid to the far wall of the postablation lesion and any margin in close proximity to a large vessel, because these are areas likely to harbor residual disease (Fig. 6) [69].

Follow-up ablation findings are much more complex on MR imaging than CT because signal charac-

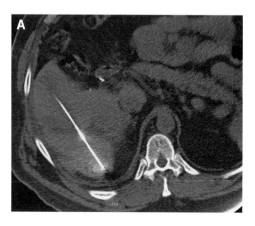 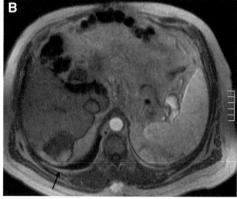

Fig. 6. (*A*) Under CT guidance, RFA is performed by a right lateral approach. (*B*) T1-weighted contrast-enhanced image 2 months following RFA demonstrates residual nodular tumor involving the far wall of the treated lesion (*arrow*).

teristics of the tumor and surrounding tissue reflect the underlying cellular composition [64]. Evaluation for recurrent tumor is done predominantly with T2-weighted images and postgadolinium T1-weighted images. Coagulated tissue appears low signal on T2-weighted images because of reduced protein density from the thermal injury [64,71]. The central ablation zone should appear dark on T2-weighted images. Slightly increased T2-signal may be seen, however, and should not be considered diagnostic of residual tumor [65,71,72]. T1-weighted images may be heterogeneous but tend to have increased signal intensity because of hemorrhage and high protein content (Fig. 7) [64,65,71]. Just as with CT, a thin rim of marginal enhancement may be seen with MR imaging after contrast administration. This can persist for several months because it represents granulation tissue and fibrosis. Asymmetric thickening or nodular

enhancement should be considered abnormal [71], however, and the combination of abnormal T2-signal with corresponding enhancement is 100% specific for residual tumor [71].

Results

When evaluating the results of RFA in the liver, both technical success and impact on survival should be considered. There are numerous reports documenting the immediate technical success in treating focal liver lesions with RFA. Curley and coworkers [73] published one of the earlier series evaluating the degree of necrosis of both hepatomas and hepatic metastases (median diameter 3.4 cm) in 123 patients following RFA. The investigators reported complete necrosis in all lesions on follow-up imaging (15-month average follow-up); an ablative site recur-

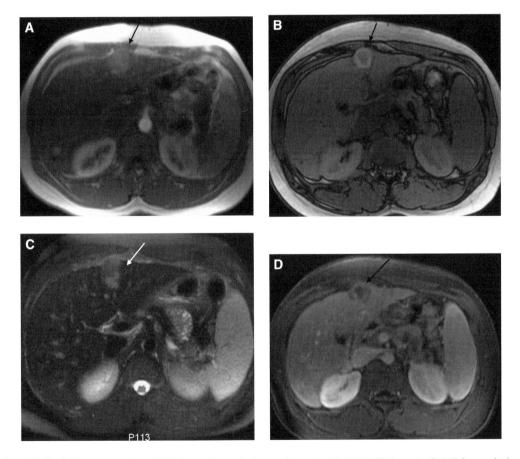

Fig. 7. (*A*) Pre-RFA contrast-enhanced MR image demonstrating a subcapsular left lobe HCC (*arrow*). (*B*) MR image obtained 2 months following RFA out-of-phase imaging demonstrates a thick rim of high signal, indicative of blood products (*arrow*). (*C*) Half-Fourier single-shot turbo spin-echo images obtained at same time demonstrates high signal within treatment bed (*arrow*). (*D*) Contrast-enhanced imaging demonstrates thick rim of high signal, correlating with blood products seen on precontrasted images, and no enhancement indicative of residual tumor (*arrow*).

rence rate of 1.8%; and the development of meta-static disease in 28%. Rossi and coworkers [74,75] demonstrated 95% and 91% complete necrosis rates for small HCC following RFA, but with recurrence rates of 41% and 29%, respectively. Although initial technical success is promising for these small lesions, recurrence rates are high, reflecting the persistent underlying liver disease or systemic disease process.

The immediate technical success of RFA for larger lesions is less encouraging. A recent study by Chen and coworkers [59] reported a complete ablation rate of 87.6% for lesions greater than 3.5 cm by using multiple, carefully placed, overlapping burns. An-other study documented a 100% complete necrosis rate for lesions less than 3 cm in diameter, which dropped to 57% for lesions larger than 5 cm [76]. In another study, complete necrosis rates fell to 48% when treating lesions over 3 cm in diameter, and often required multiple treatment sessions [44]. To enhance coagulation volumes, combined therapies have been used in these patients with larger tumors, and reports of complete tumor kill for lesions up to 12 cm have been reported [33]. The development of recurrent disease, however, remains problematic.

There is adequate evidence that RFA can con-sistently result in complete necrosis of small lesions, with more variable response following treatment of medium to large lesions. Reports investigating RFA and impact on survival are less readily available. A recent prospective study evaluated patient survival following locoregional therapies for HCC, and found that patients with complete remission had a signifi-cantly better long-term survival than those without [77]. A second study specifically evaluated the ef-fect of RFA on patient survival [78]. In this report, 282 patients with early, nonoperable HCC were treated with percutaneous ablation. Initial complete response was achieved in 70% of patients. Overall survival rates were 87%, 51%, and 27% at 1, 3, and 5 years, respectively, which compares favorably with surgical resection. Multivariate analysis demon-strated that Child-Pugh score and complete necrosis of the lesion were independent predictors of survival, indicating the importance of complete tumor eradi-cation at time of treatment.

With respect to colorectal metastases, three recent papers have evaluated RFA and survival. A single center study demonstrated 3- and 5-year survival rates of 42.9% and 19.2% following thermal ablation, which compared favorably with the 43.5% and 32.1% survival rates following surgical resection [79]. Gillams and Lees [9] reported their prospective series of RFA in 167 patients with colorectal metastases who were either nonsurgical candidates or had

refused surgery. For patients with ≤ 5 lesions with a maximum diameter of 5 cm or less and no extra-hepatic disease, the 5-year survival from the time of diagnosis was 30%, which compared favorably with a 5-year surgical survival of 32% (even more notable because many of these patients were not surgical candidates). Berber and coworkers [80] evaluated 135 patients with nonresectable colon metastases who underwent laparoscopic RFA. The median Kaplan-Meier survival was 28.9 months, improved from the historical median survival of 5 to 10 months if no treatment is initiated. The study identified a carcino-embryonic antigen level of less than 200 ng/mL and dominant lesion less than 3 cm to be significant factors with respect to survival. A trend was identified toward improved survival in patients with one to three tumors in comparison with patients with more than three tumors, but this did not reach significance. Liver tumor size larger than 5 cm was a significant predictor of mortality, demonstrating a 2.5-fold increased risk of death compared with patients with tumors measuring less than 3 cm.

Complications

The overall complication rate for RFA is low. Immediately following the procedure, the patient may experience a postablation syndrome [81]. This con-sists of symptoms including pain, low-grade fever, and malaise. It is typically self-limiting and may per-sist anywhere from a few days to several weeks. The syndrome is generally in proportion to the amount of tumor ablated, and can be managed conservatively. If symptoms worsen over time or the patient develops high fever, a more serious complication should be considered. Development of an asymptomatic right-sided pleural effusion is also not uncommon, and usually resolves without incident.

A recent single center study evaluated complica-tion rates associated with 1000 RFA treatments in 2140 hepatomas affecting 664 patients, and demon-strated a major and minor complication rate of 4% and 1.7%, respectively [82]. Major complications included intraperitoneal hemorrhage, hepatic infarc-tion, hepatic abscess formation, intestinal perforation, and bile peritonitis. With respect to hepatic abscess formation, it is interesting to note that patients who had undergone prior bilioenteric anastomosis or sphincterotomy were not included in the study group. Additionally, all patients received preprocedural and postprocedural antibiotics, which were continued if the patient remained febrile. Fifteen cases of tumor track seeding were identified during the study period. Minor complications included self-limited hemobilia, needle entry site skin burn, portal vein thrombosis, and biloma formation. There were no treatment-related deaths in this series.

A larger, multicenter study investigated RFA-related complications associated with treating 3554 lesions [50]. This study reported an overall lower major complication rate of 2.5%, but included within this 2.5% were six patient deaths (0.3%) attributed to nontarget thermal injury, hemorrhage following tumor rupture, liver failure following the development of biliary stenosis, peritonitis, and septic shock. Other nonfatal major complications included massive intraperitoneal hemorrhage, biliary injury, and hepatic abscess formation. In this study, hepatic abscess formation was associated with patients who had undergone prior bilioenteric anastomoses, and occurred even after intravenous antibiotics had been administered. Delayed tumor seeding was identified in 0.5% of patients. Minor complications were seen in an additional 4.7%, and included grounding pad injuries. Other reported complications have included main portal vein thrombosis (usually associated with arresting portal vein flow during RFA) and asymptomatic vascular occlusion.

Summary

Unresectable liver lesions caused by either primary malignancies or metastatic disease carry a dismal prognosis. As such, the use of locoregional hepatic treatments has become extremely popular in clinical practice and as a topic of much research. There is a large body of data indicating that RFA can reliably treat tumors less than 3 cm in diameter. The modality by itself is less effective, however, when applied to larger tumors. Additionally, there are only a few scattered reports indicating that RFA improves survival in patients with either HCC or metastatic disease. Large controlled, randomized, clinical trials evaluating improved locoregional techniques including RFA, combined techniques, and effect on long-term patient survival are necessary to determine what is truly beneficial for the patient. In the meantime, proper patient selection, careful preoperative evaluation, and appropriate planning can maximize patient outcome while minimizing complications.

References

[1] Patt CH, Thuluvath PJ. Role of liver transplantation in the management of hepatocellular carcinoma. J Vasc Interv Radiol 2002;13:S205–10.

[2] McGahan J, Dodd G. Radiofrequency ablation of the liver: current status. AJR Am J Roentgenol 2001;176:3–16.

[3] Cha C, DeMatto RP, Blumgart LH. Surgery and ablative therapy for hepatocellular carcinoma. J Clin Gastroenterol 2002;35(Suppl 2):130–7.

[4] Befeler AS, DiBisceglie AM. Hepatocellular carcinoma: diagnosis and treatment. Gastroenterology 2002;122:1609–19.

[5] Choti MA. Surgical management of hepatocellular carcinoma: resection and ablation. J Vasc Interv Radiol 2002;13:S197–203.

[6] Choi D, Lim HK, Kim MJ, et al. Recurrent hepatocellular carcinoma: percutaneous radiofrequency ablation after hepatectomy. Radiology 2004;230:135–41.

[7] Fisher R, Maluf D, Cotterell AH, et al. Non-resective ablation therapy for hepatocellular carcinoma: effectiveness measured by intention-to-treat and dropout from liver transplant waiting list. Clin Transplant 2004;18:502–12.

[8] Tsalis K, Vasiliadis K, Christoforidis E, et al. Current treatment of colorectal liver metastases. Tech Coloproctol 2004;8:S174–6.

[9] Gillams AR, Lees WR. Radio-frequency ablation of colorectal liver metastases in 167 patients. Eur Radiol 2004;14:2261–7.

[10] Fong Y, Fortner J, Sun RL, et al. Clinical score for predicting recurrence after hepatic resection for metastatic colorectal cancer: analysis of 1001 consecutive cases. Ann Surg 1999;230:309–21.

[11] Solbiati L, Livraghi T, Goldberg SN, et al. Percutaneous radio-frequency ablation of hepatic metastases from colorectal cancer: long-term results in 117 patients. Radiology 2001;221:159–66.

[12] de Baere T, Elias D, Dromain C, et al. Radiofrequency ablation of 100 hepatic metastases with a mean follow-up of more than 1 year. AJR Am J Roentgenol 2000;175:1619–25.

[13] Rhim H, Goldberg SN, Dodd 3rd GD, et al. Essential techniques for successful radiofrequency thermal ablation of malignant hepatic tumors. Radiographics 2001;21:517–39.

[14] Kruskal JB, Oliver B, Huertas JC, et al. Dynamic intrahepatic flow and cellular alterations during radiofrequency ablation of liver tissue in mice. J Vasc Interv Radiol 2001;12:1193–201.

[15] McGahan JP, Brock JM, Tesluk H, et al. Hepatic ablation using radiofrequency electrocautery in the animal model. Invest Radiol 1990;25:267–70.

[16] Rossi S, Fornari F, Pathies C. Thermal lesions induced by 480 KHz localized current field in guinea pig and pig liver. Tumori 1990;76:54–7.

[17] Goldberg SN, Gazelle GS, Mueller PR. Thermal ablation therapy for focal malignancy: a unified approach to underlying principles, techniques, and diagnostic imaging guidance. AJR Am J Roentgenol 2000;174:323–31.

[18] Pennes H. Analysis of tissue and arterial blood tem-

peratures in the resting human forearm. J Appl Physiol 1998;1:93–122.

[19] LeVeen R. Laser hyperthermia and radiofrequency ablation of hepatic lesions. Semin Interv Radiol 1997; 14:313–24.

[20] de Baere T, Denys A, Wood BJ, et al. Radiofrequency liver ablation: experimental comparative study of water-cooled versus expandable systems. AJR Am J Roentgenol 2001;176:187–92.

[21] Gebauer B, Gaffke G, Hunerbein M, et al. Flexible applicator systems for radiofrequency ablation (RFA) hepatic tumors [abstract]. Rofo Fortschr Geb Rontgenstr Neuen Bildgeb 2003;175:1720–3.

[22] Pereira PL, Trubenbach J, Schenk M, et al. Radiofrequency ablation: in vivo comparison of four commercially available devices in pig livers. Radiology 2004;232:482–90.

[23] Rossi S, Garbagnati F, Rosa L, et al. Radiofrequency thermal ablation for treatment of hepatocellular carcinoma. Int J Oncol 2002;7:225–35.

[24] Denys AL, de Baere T, Kuoch V, et al. Radiofrequency tissue ablation of the liver: in vivo and ex vivo experiments with four different systems. Eur Radiol 2003;13:2346–52.

[25] Goldberg SN, Ahmed M, Gazelle GS. Radio-frequency thermal ablation with NaCl solution injection: effect of electrical conductivity on tissue heating and coagulation-phantom and porcine liver study. Radiology 2001;219:157–65.

[26] Miao Y, Ni Y, Yu J, et al. An ex vivo study on radiofrequency tissue ablation: increased lesion size by using an "expandable-wet" electrode. Eur Radiol 2001;11:1841–7.

[27] Horkan C, Goldberg SN. History, principles, and techniques of radiofrequency ablation. Semin Interv Radiol 2003;20:253–68.

[28] Lu DS, Raman SS, Vodopich DJ, et al. Effect of vessel size on creation of hepatic radiofrequency lesions in pigs: assessment of the "heat sink" effect. AJR Am J Roentgenol 2002;178:47–51.

[29] Kurokohchi K, Masaki T, Miyauchi Y. Efficacy of combination therapies of percutaneous or laparoscopic ethanol-lipiodol injection and radiofrequency ablation. Int J Oncol 2004;25:1737–43.

[30] Goldberg SN, Hahn PF, Halpern EF, et al. Radiofrequency tissue ablation: effect of pharmacologic modulation of blood flow on coagulation diameter. Radiology 1998;209:761–7.

[31] Patterson EJ, Scudamore CH, Owen DA, et al. Radiofrequency ablation of porcine liver in vivo: effects of blood flow and treatment time on lesion size. Ann Surg 1998;227:559–65.

[32] Rossi S, Garbagnati F, Lencioni R, et al. Percutaneous radio-frequency thermal ablation of nonresectable hepatocellular carcinoma after occlusion of tumor blood supply. Radiology 2000;217:119–26.

[33] Yamakado K, Nakatsuka A, Ohmori S, et al. Radiofrequency ablation combined with chemoembolization in hepatocellular carcinoma: treatment response based on tumor size and morphology. J Vasc Interv Radiol 2002;13:1225–32.

[34] Lee JM, Lee YH, Kim SW, et al. Combined treatment of radiofrequency ablation and acetic acid injection: an in vivo feasibility study in rabbit liver. Eur Radiol 2004;14(7):1303–10.

[35] Kurokohchi K, Watanabe S, Masaki T, et al. Combined use of percutaneous ethanol injection and radiofrequency ablation for the effective treatment of hepatocellular carcinoma. Int J Oncol 2002;21:841–6.

[36] Kurokohchi K, Watanabe S, Masaki T, et al. Combination therapy of percutaneous ethanol injection and radiofrequency ablation against hepatocellular carcinomas difficult to treat. Int J Oncol 2002;21:611–5.

[37] Ahmed M, Weinstein J, Liu Z, et al. Image-guided percutaneous chemical and radiofrequency tumor ablation in an animal model. J Vasc Interv Radiol 2003;14: 1045–52.

[38] Goldberg SN, Saldinger PF, Gazelle GS, et al. Percutaneous tumor ablation: increased necrosis with combined radiofrequency ablation and intratumoral doxorubicin injection in a rat breast tumor model. Radiology 2001;220:420–7.

[39] Goldberg SN, Kamel IR, Kruskal JB, et al. Radiofrequency ablation of hepatic tumors: increased tumor destruction with adjuvant liposomal doxorubicin therapy. AJR Am J Roentgenol 2002;179:93–101.

[40] Hori T, Murakami T, Oi H, et al. Sensitivity in detection of hypervascular hepatocellular carcinoma by helical CT with intra-arterial injection of contrast medium, and by helical CT and MR imaging with intravenous injection of contrast medium. Acta Radiol 1998;39:144–51.

[41] de Lange EE, Mugler 3rd JP, Gay SB, et al. Focal liver disease: comparison of breath-hold T1-weighted MP-GRE MR imaging and contrast-enhanced CT: lesion detection, localization, and characterization. Radiology 1996;200:465–73.

[42] Yamada S, Yamashita Y, Mitsuzaki K, et al. Small hepatocellular carcinoma in patients with chronic liver damage: prospective comparison of detection with dynamic MR imaging and helical CT of the whole liver. Radiology 1996;200:79–84.

[43] Livraghi T, Goldberg SN, Lazzaroni S, et al. Small hepatocellular carcinoma: treatment with radiofrequency ablation versus ethanol injection. Radiology 1999;210:655–61.

[44] Livraghi T, Goldberg SN, Lazzaroni S, et al. Hepatocellular carcinoma: radio-frequency ablation of medium and large lesions. Radiology 2000;214:761–8.

[45] Mazzaferro V, Battiston C, Perrone S. Radiofrequency ablation of small hepatocellular carcinoma in cirrhotic patients awaiting liver transplantation: a prospective study. Ann Surg 2004;240:900–9.

[46] Hori T, Nagata K, Hasuike S. Risk factors for the local recurrence of hepatocellular carcinoma after a single session of percutaneous radiofrequency ablation. J Gastroenterol 2003;38:977–81.

[47] Chopra D, Dodd 3rd GD, Chanin MP, et al. Radio-

frequency ablation of hepatic tumors adjacent to the gallbladder: feasibility and safety. AJR Am J Roentgenol 2003;180:697–701.

[48] Poon R, Ng KK, Lam CK, et al. Radiofrequency ablation for subcapsular hepatocellular carcinoma. Ann Surg Oncol 2004;11:281–9.

[49] de Baere T, Risse O, Kuoch V, et al. Adverse events during radiofrequency treatment of 582 hepatic tumors. AJR Am J Roentgenol 2003;181:695–700.

[50] Livraghi T, Solbiati L, Meloni MF, et al. Treatment of focal liver tumors with percutaneous radio-frequency ablation: complications encountered in a multicenter study. Radiology 2003;226:441–51.

[51] Lu DS, Raman SS, Vodopich DJ, et al. Influence of large peritumoral vessels on outcome of radiofrequency ablation of liver tumors. J Vasc Interv Radiol 2003;14:1267–74.

[52] Dupuy DE, Goldberg SN. Image-guided radiofrequency tumor ablation: challenges and opportunities-Part I. J Vasc Interv Radiol 2001;12:1135–48.

[53] Sato M, Watanabe Y, Tokui K, et al. CT-guided treatment of ultrasonically invisible hepatocellular carcinoma. Am J Gastroenterol 2000;95:2102–6.

[54] Zheng X-H, Guan YS, Zhou XP. Detection of hypervascular hepatocellular carcinoma: comparison of multi-detector CT with digital subtraction angiography and Lipiodol CT. World J Gastroenterol 2005;11: 200–3.

[55] Numata K, Isozaki T, Ozawi Y, et al. Percutaneous ablation therapy guided by contrast-enhanced sonography for patients with hepatocellular carcinoma. AJR Am J Roentgenol 2003;180:143–9.

[56] Mahnken AH, Bueker A, Spuentrup E, et al. MR-guided radiofrequency ablation of hepatic malignancies at 1.5 T: initial results. J Magn Reson Imaging 2004;19:342–8.

[57] Shibata T, Buecker A, Spuentrup E, et al. Cholangitis and liver abscess after percutaneous ablation therapy for liver tumors: incidence and risk factors. J Vasc Interv Radiol 2003;14:1535–42.

[58] Dodd 3rd GD, Soulen MC, Kane RA, et al. Minimally invasive treatment of malignant hepatic tumors: at the threshold of a major breakthrough. Radiographics 2000;20:9–27.

[59] Chen M-H, Yang W, Yan K. Large liver tumors: protocol for radiofrequency ablation and its clinical application in 110 patients: mathematic model, overlapping mode, and electrode placement process. Radiology 2004;232:260–71.

[60] Leyendecker JR, Dodd 3rd GD, Halff GA, et al. Sonographically observed echogenic response during intraoperative radiofrequency ablation of cirrhotic livers: pathologic correlation. AJR Am J Roentgenol 2002;178:1147–51.

[61] Cioni D, Lencioni R, Rossi S, et al. Radiofrequency thermal ablation of hepatocellular carcinoma: using contrast-enhanced harmonic power Doppler sonography to assess treatment outcome. AJR Am J Roentgenol 2001;177:783–8.

[62] Goldberg N, Dupuy DE. Image-guided radiofrequency tumor ablation: challenges and opportunities–part I. J Vasc Interv Radiol 2001;12:1021–32.

[63] Raman SS, Lu DS, Vodopich DJ. Creation of radiofrequency lesions in a porcine model: correlation with sonography, CT, and histopathology. AJR Am J Roentgenol 2000;175:1253–8.

[64] Masashi T, Tsuda M, Rikimaru H, et al. Time-related changes of radiofrequency ablation lesion in the normal rabbit liver: findings of magnetic resonance imaging and histopathology. Invest Radiol 2003;38: 525–31.

[65] Limanond P, Zimmerman P, Raman SS, et al. Interpretation of CT and MRI after radiofrequency ablation of hepatic malignancies. AJR Am J Roentgenol 2003; 181:1635–40.

[66] Anderson GS, Brinkmann F, Soulen MC, et al. FDG positron emission tomography in the surveillance of hepatic tumors treated with radiofrequency ablation. Clin Nucl Med 2003;28:192–7.

[67] Donckier V, Van Laethem JL, Goldman S, et al. [F-18] fluorodeoxyglucose positron emission tomography as a tool for early recognition of incomplete tumor destruction after radiofrequency ablation for liver metastases. J Surg Oncol 2003;84:215–23.

[68] Goldberg SN, Gazelle GS, Compton CC. Treatment of intrahepatic malignancy with radiofrequency ablation: radiologic-pathologic correlation. Cancer 2000;88: 2452–63.

[69] Catalano O, Esposito M, Nunziata A, et al. Multiphase helical CT findings after percutaneous ablation procedures for hepatocellular carcinoma. Abdom Imaging 2000;25:607–14.

[70] Chopra S, Dodd 3rd GD, Chintapalli KN, et al. Tumor recurrence after radiofrequency thermal ablation of hepatic tumors: spectrum of findings on dual-phase contrast-enhanced CT. AJR Am J Roentgenol 2001; 177:381–7.

[71] Guan Y-S, Sun L, Zhou XP, et al. Hepatocellular carcinoma treated with interventional procedures: CT and MRI follow-up. World J Gastroenterol 2004;10: 3543–8.

[72] Sironi S, Livraghi T, Meloni F, et al. Small hepatocellular carcinoma treated with percutaneous RF ablation: MR imaging follow-up. AJR Am J Roentgenol 1999; 173:1225–9.

[73] Curley SA, Izzo F, Delrio P, et al. Radiofrequency ablation of unresectable primary and metastatic hepatic malignancies: results in 123 patients. Ann Surg 1999; 230:1–8.

[74] Rossi S, Di Stasi M, Buscarini E, et al. Percutaneous radiofrequency interstitial thermal ablation in the treatment of small hepatocellular carcinoma. Cancer J Sci Am 1995;1:73.

[75] Rossi S, Buscarini E, Gabagnati F. Percutaneous treatment of small hepatic tumors by an expandable RF needle electrode. AJR Am J Roentgenol 1998;170: 1015–22.

[76] Ruzzenente A, Manzoni GD, Molfetta M, et al. Rapid

progression of hepatocellular carcinoma after radio-frequency ablation. World J Gastroenterol 2004;10: 1137–40.

[77] Huo TI, Huang YH, Wu JC, et al. Induction of complete tumor necrosis may reduce intrahepatic metastasis and prolong survival in patients with hepatocellular carcinoma undergoing locoregional therapy: a prospective study. Ann Surg Oncol 2004;15:775–80.

[78] Sala M, Llovet JM, Vilana R, et al. Initial response to percutaneous ablation predicts survival in patients with hepatocellular carcinoma. Hepatology 2004;40: 1352–60.

[79] Ji Z-L, Peng SY, Yuan AJ, et al. Hepatic resection for metastasis from colorectal cancer. Tech Coloproctol 2004;8:S47–9.

[80] Berber E, Pelley R, Siperstein AE. Predictors of survival after radiofrequency thermal ablation of colorectal cancer metastases to the liver: a prospective study. J Clin Oncol 2005;31:1358–64.

[81] Goldberg S, Charboneau JW, Dodd 3rd GD, et al. Image-guided tumor ablation: proposal for standardization of terms and reporting criteria. Radiology 2003; 228:335–45.

[82] Ryosuke T, Shiina S, Teratini T, et al. Percutaneous radiofrequency ablation for hepatocellular carcinoma. Cancer 2005.

ELSEVIER
SAUNDERS

Radiol Clin N Am 43 (2005) 915–927

RADIOLOGIC
CLINICS
of North America

Pre-, Peri-, and Posttreatment Imaging of Liver Lesions

Larissa Braga, MD, PhD[a], Ulrich Guller, MD, MHSc[b],
Richard C. Semelka, MD[a],*

[a]Department of Radiology, School of Medicine, University of North Carolina at Chapel Hill, 101 Manning Drive, CB 7510,
Chapel Hill, NC 27599–7510, USA
[b]Divisions of General Surgery and Surgical Research, Department of Surgery, University of Basel, Spitalstrasse 21,
4031 Basel, Switzerland

Major recent advances and technical progress in liver surgery and transplantation have been possible, in part because of improved understanding of the anatomy of the liver provided by modern imaging methods. Moreover, small asymptomatic tumors, frequently undetected in the past, can now be visualized. The increasing detection of early stage liver malignancies with current-generation imaging modalities has fostered the concurrent development of new, less invasive therapeutic approaches to improve patient survival.

Surgical resection with negative (R0) tumor margins remains the first choice in the treatment of liver malignancies. This curative approach is only possible, however, in about 5% to 25% of patients [1–3]. Although liver resection is predominantly performed in patients with liver metastases from colon cancer, current preliminary studies have reported promising results in breast cancer patients with liver metastases [4,5].

As an alternative or supplement to surgery, a variety of chemotherapy regimens play an important role in the management of liver metastases. New types and classes of chemotherapeutic agents, some of them still investigational, may increase the life expectancy of patients with liver malignancies. There is a variety of different chemotherapeutic agents and their mechanisms of action are complex. Recent studies have suggested that the antiangiogenic effect of some of these agents could in part be responsible for particular posttreatment imaging features of liver malignancies, such as hemangioma-like appearances [6,7].

Transcatheter arterial chemoembolization therapy is based on the premise that hypervascular malignant tumors are supplied mainly by branches of the hepatic artery. The catheter is selectively introduced into the hepatic artery and chemotherapeutic agents along with embolic substances are instilled. This has not only a cytotoxic effect on malignant cells but also causes obliteration of the arteries that feed the tumor [8,9]. Among all liver malignancies, metastases from colon cancer, neuroendocrine tumors, and hepatocellular carcinomas (HCC) are most commonly treated with this approach [10–14].

If curative resection of liver malignancies is not possible, ablative therapies are the second choice in the therapeutic algorithm. Although long-term results are still lacking, it is established that ablative therapies are associated with low postinterventional morbidity and mortality, and low cost compared with resection [15,16]. Ablative therapies provide direct tumor destruction with mild damage to the surrounding parenchyma. The manner through which the tumor is ablated can be classified as either chemical or thermal ablation. Chemical ablation refers to the use of ethanol injection. Thermal ablation can be subcategorized as follow: by heat (radiofrequency [RF] ablation, microwave ablation, laser ablation); and by cold (cryoablation) [17]. Among all these therapeutic options, RF ablation seems to be the most promising approach [18–20].

---

* Corresponding author.
E-mail address: richsem@med.unc.edu (R.C. Semelka).

RF ablation, cryoablation, microwave ablation, and laser ablation have mainly been performed in the setting of HCC and metastases from colon cancer [18–24]. Recent investigations, however, have reported the use of these ablative methods in patients with metastases from neck, breast, pancreas, and stomach cancer [23,25]. Ethanol ablation is performed predominantly in the treatment of HCC [18,19]. The primary goal of ablative therapies is curative [8]; however, some of the procedures are performed to alleviate clinical symptoms, to obtain tumor regression that enables subsequent surgical resection [13,23,26], or to lengthen patient survival.

Liver transplantation has been shown to be an alternative therapeutic approach in cirrhotic patients with HCC, if liver resection is not an option because of a limited hepatic reserve. Recent investigations report the results of liver transplantation in patients with metastases from a variety of primary sites [27,28]. The shortage of liver donors and resulting long waiting list often necessitate that first patients undergo ablative therapies as a stabilizing or temporizing measure, however, and then as second step, liver transplantation.

Pretreatment imaging

Detection and characterization

Among all diagnostic methods, MR provides the most accurate imaging and has the highest sensitivity in the depiction and characterization of focal liver lesions. The superiority of MR imaging is achieved by the combination of multiplanar T1- and T2-weighted images and serial dynamic imaging after gadolinium contrast administration [29–31].

Number and size

The information regarding the number and size of hepatic tumors is crucial in the planning of liver resection, ablative procedures, and liver transplantation. These determine various factors, such as type of resection; ablative therapy, chemotherapy, or combination; type of the probe; the number of sessions required to achieve an adequate ablation; or the volume of ethanol instilled in the ethanol-ablation procedure. Moreover, it has been suggested that patients eligible for ablative therapy must have one hepatic malignancy ≤ 5 cm or as many as three lesions each ≤ 3 cm [32]. Successful ablation is more likely in small tumors compared with larger ones

[33,34]. Hasegawa and coworkers [33] reported that HCC ≤ 1.5 cm had a lower risk of local recurrence than larger HCC after ethanol ablation therapy. Large tumors may be suitable for cryoablation therapy or for a combined therapeutic approach [22,23,35,36].

The indication for applying systemic chemotherapy or transcatheter chemoembolization therapy is not affected by the size or the number of hepatic lesions. Both therapies can be performed even if large or multiple malignancies are scattered throughout the liver parenchyma [22].

Anatomic localization

Tumors should be localized on imaging examinations according to the Couinaud criteria [37], which facilitates their identification during resection, intervention, or other treatment procedures. Small tumors, which are detected by CT or MR examinations, may not always be visualized by ultrasound, which is the main imaging method used in the guidance of ablative therapies. Moreover, the knowledge of tumor location helps the interventional radiologist or surgeon to predict complications or side effects that may occur after therapy.

Pain is commonly reported after ablative therapy when the tumor is in close proximity to the diaphragm, liver capsule, gallbladder, or main portal vein [38]. Patients with superficial lesions near the diaphragm are more likely to have pleural effusion, pneumothorax, and hemothorax after tumor ablation.

It is also critical to report the proximity of the tumor to important structures, such as main vessels, gallbladder, and central bile ducts, because this impacts the success of treatment. For instance, RF ablation is less likely to be successful in tumors that are located near large vessels. This can be explained by a decrease of the temperature inside the tumor caused by nearby blood flow, preventing the intense heat required to cause cell death, a phenomenon called "heat-sink effect" [38,39]. Furthermore, it is recognizes that ablation of tumors in close proximity to gallbladder and central bile ducts is associated with damage to these structures resulting in considerable postoperative morbidity [32,38].

Tumor vascularity

Tumor vascularity and pattern of vascularity also have predictive value to determine the type of treatment procedure to which the disease is likely to respond. It has been shown that small, uniformly vascular tumors are more likely to show good response to chemoembolization than larger, heterogeneously vascular, or hypovascular tumors [40,41]. As new chemotherapeutic agents with different biologic properties continue to be developed, tumor vascularity as shown on MR imaging may also permit triaging patients to various regimens.

Presence of venous tumor invasion or extrahepatic disease

Tumor thrombus in main vessels or extrahepatic metastases are usually contraindications for liver resection, ablative therapies, and liver transplantation [35]. Portal vein thrombosis is often seen in the setting of large HCC [40].

During treatment

Ultrasound is the most frequently used imaging method to guide ablative therapies. The low cost, feasibility, absence of radiation, and real-time data acquisition of ultrasound make it the preferred imaging method among interventional radiologists and surgeons. Preliminary studies that have used MR imaging to guide ablative therapies have been reported [42,43], and the results seem promising. MR imaging provides better contrast between structures and background parenchyma than CT or ultrasound, and consequently more anatomic detail [16]. This is crucial information because tumor boundary must be defined accurately before and during ablative therapies to achieve complete tumor treatment.

Intraoperative ultrasound represents an important tool for surgeons to perform liver resection or to guide ablative therapies, such as cryoablation. In addition, intraoperative ultrasound facilitates the accurate definition of tumor edges and the relationship with anatomic structures. It is critically important to detect all tumor masses because this allows adequate surgical or interventional removal and destruction, and improves patient survival.

Imaging evaluation after treatment

Size

Tumor size can be well assessed on unenhanced T1-weighted MR images. T1-weighted images acquired before and immediately after gadolinium administration also permit distinction between lesional and perilesional enhancement. Lesional enhancement refers to enhancement within the tumor, whereas perilesional enhancement is enhancement beyond the tumor margin. This distinction may have importance in the assessment of tumor response after systemic chemotherapy in patients with hypovascular liver metastases (see below).

Systemic chemotherapy

Tumor response following systemic chemotherapy, based on the change in number and size of the tumors, is described according to World Health Organization criteria: (1) complete response, (2) partial response, (3) stable disease, and (4) disease progression. Decrease in tumor size represents the standard imaging sign used for assessing effectiveness of systemic chemotherapy. It has been reported, however, that some tumors undergo complete necrosis during chemotherapy without diminishing in size [44]. This is particularly true in the setting of cirrhotic livers, which may lack the cellular constituents' ability to remove necrotic debris that results in a prolonged healing process [45,46].

Ablative therapies

Whether or not tumor ablation is successful can be predicted by evaluating the size of the necrotic cavity postprocedure. The necrotic cavity must exceed the tumor margins by 0.5 to 1 cm [16]. The ablation of adjacent healthy liver parenchyma enables the eradication of microscopic tumor in the tumor boundary. Achieving a wide ablation margin is especially important if the tumor borders are ill-defined [16]. A recent study demonstrated that 80% (four out of five) of the cases that showed similar dimensions of the pretreatment tumor and posttreatment necrotic cavity had residual tumor at histopathologic analysis, which was not revealed on imaging studies [15].

If the treatment is successful, the ablated zone either remains with similar dimensions as immediately posttherapy, or may regress in size [17,47]. The pace at which the ablated zone shrinks after intervention depends on the therapy used and the presence or absence of underlying liver disease. For instance, tumors ablated with ethanol tend to shrink faster than tumors treated with RF ablation [47,48]. It has been proposed that the measurement of the tumor and the ablated zone should be made using tridimensional imaging because this enables a more accurate assessment of the success of the ablation method [17].

MR imaging findings of successful treatment

Liver resection

Surgical resection causes damage in the healthy liver parenchyma along the resection margin. The injury in the hepatic parenchyma is reflected by focal areas of edema and granulation tissue. By imaging, the focal areas can acquire different shapes but linear circular, oval, or serpiginous are most commonly described [49]. On MR imaging, the focal areas are characterized by high signal intensity on T2-weighted images, low signal intensity on T1-weighted images, and homogeneously mild to moderate enhancement on arterial-dominant phase images that fade away toward background isointensity on interstitial phase images [49,50]. These nonneoplastic areas tend to resolve 3 to 5 months after intervention [40,49].

Systemic chemotherapy

It has been suggested that after 2 weeks of good response, there is a decrease in both tumor size and vascularity, associated with an increase in central necrosis (Fig. 1) [51]. On T2-weighted images, early in the course of therapy responsive tumors exhibit high signal intensity reflecting high extracellular water content caused by necrosis; but progressively they show decrease in signal intensity caused by cellular dehydration and reduction in vascularity [6,41,52,53].

On MR imaging, the vascularity of liver tumors can be assessed using dynamic serial gadolinium-enhanced imaging. Liver tumors can be classified as hypervascular or hypovascular based on the extent of enhancement on arterial-dominant phase images. Previous MR studies correlated the vascularity of liver metastases with tumor response after systemic chemotherapy [6,7]. One report showed a correlation between decreased tumor size after treatment and diminution of tumor vascularization [7]. Another study associated tumor hypovascularity with successful treatment, correlated with histopathologic analysis [6]. Tumor vascularity may also correlate with patient outcome. In a recent study [54], patients who had persistently hypervascular liver metastases from breast cancer following systemic chemotherapy demonstrated a higher probability of having disease progression than patients in whom liver metastases became hypovascular.

Perilesional enhancement is defined as enhancement that occurs beyond the tumor confines and extends into surrounding hepatic parenchyma, and is best appreciated on arterial-dominant phase images [55]. Histopathologic analysis demonstrated that perilesional enhancement on MR imaging correlated with the presence of peritumoral desmoplastic reaction, peritumoral inflammation, and vascular proliferation [56]. Although perilesional enhancement is most often appreciated in hypovascular liver metastases (eg, from colon cancer), it may also be observed with hypervascular liver metastases (eg, from breast cancer) [56]. Chemotherapeutic agents reduce tumor growth rate, inflammatory changes, and tumor angiogenesis, all of which may contribute to a decrease in perilesional enhancement [57]. It has been shown that a decrease in the extent of perilesional enhancement after systemic chemotherapy reflects a positive tumor response [6].

In the long term, tumors that respond to systemic chemotherapy may either disappear or become fibrotic. Fibrotic areas appear as irregular, angular-shaped foci often associated with distortion of adjacent hepatic parenchyma and capsule retraction, if the treated-tumor is superficially located. Mature fibrosis appears as isointensity or low signal intensity on T2-weighted images and moderately low signal intensity on T1-weighted images. On initial postcontrast images mature fibrosis exhibits negligible enhancement, but tends to enhance progressively on interstitial phase images.

Transcatheter arterial chemoembolization

Tumors that are adequately treated by transcatheter arterial chemoembolization are usually replaced by necrosis. Because of the concomitant arterial occlusion substantial tissue fluid is not present. As a result, on MR imaging the necrotic area appears moderately low to isointense in signal intensity on T2-weighted images reflecting the low fluid content, which is a distinctive appearance for lesions treated with transcatheter arterial chemoembolization. Similar to other ablative therapies the region is low signal on T1-weighted images, and shows lack of enhancement after contrast administration [41,58].

Ablation therapy

Up to 1 week after ablation, the necrotic cavity shows a wide variation from high to low signal intensity on T1- and T2-weighted images. The signal intensity on T1-weighted images is determined by the stage of the hemorrhage, whereas the signal intensity on T2-weighed images is influenced by the presence of either coagulative necrosis or liquefactive necrosis

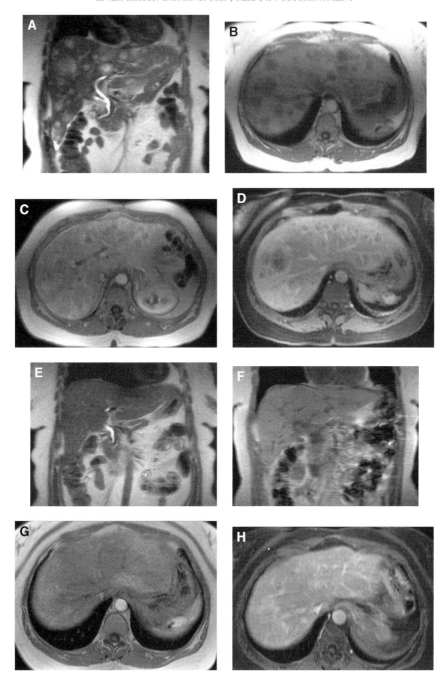

Fig. 1. Prior and after chemotherapy. Coronal T2-weighted single-shot echo-train spin-echo (SS-ETSE) (*A*), transverse T1-weighted spoiled-gradient echo (SGE) (*B*), immediate postgadolinium SGE (*C*), and 90-second fat-suppressed postgadolinium SGE (*D*) images in a patient with liver metastases from breast cancer prior chemotherapy. Coronal T2-weighted SS-ETSE (*E*), T1-weighted SGE (*F*), transverse immediate postgadolinium SGE (*G*), and 90-second fat-suppressed postgadolinium SGE (*H*) images after chemotherapy. There are multiple rounded lesions scattered throughout the hepatic parenchyma before treatment that demonstrate high signal intensity on T2-weighted image (*A*), low signal intensity on T1-weighted images (*B*), and faint ring and perilesional enhancement immediately after administration of gadolinium (*C*) that persist on late-phase images (*D*) compatible with metastases. After treatment (*E–H*) no definable lesions are identified, but patchy hepatic enhancement is apparent on early postgadolinium images (*G*).

[16,59,60]. Coagulative necrosis appears as low signal intensity and liquefactive necrosis as high signal intensity on T2-weighted images [59]. After contrast administration, the necrotic cavity shows no, or negligible, enhancement on all phases.

In the immediate postablation period, a smooth rim surrounding the necrotic cavity can be observed that shows high signal intensity on T2-weighted images and moderate to intense enhancement on arterial-dominant phase images [16,59,60]. By 1 week postprocedure the rim of enhancement generally ranges from 1 to 3 mm in thickness, but up to 5 mm may be observed [15,17]. The thickness of this rim tends to regress progressively, and the extent of enhancement on arterial-dominant phase images also diminishes, until complete disappearance generally by 6 months after ablation [16,17,40,59,61]. On hepatic arterial-dominant phase images, ill-defined perilesional enhancement is observed, reflecting inflammatory changes, which also progressively subsides, and disappears approximately 3 to 6 months following therapy.

The histopathologic analysis of the rim surrounding the necrotic cavity immediately after ablation shows intense inflammatory reaction and hemorrhage. Gradually, the inflammatory reaction and hemorrhage are replaced by granulation tissue [15,16,59]. Angiogenesis also occurs during the healing process and arises 2 to 3 days after injury, persisting for weeks to several months [62,63]. The angiogenesis in the granulation tissue is part of the healing process; however, it also provides a favorable environment for the growth of residual tumoral tissue that has not been successfully ablated [59].

The presence of air in the ablated cavity immediatcly after ablation represents a common and normal feature and tends to disappear within 1 month [61,64,65]. It has been suggested that air within the necrotic cavity originates from the process of tissue necrosis or the introduction of air bubbles along the probe during the ablation [64,65]. On MR imaging, gas bubbles appear signal void on both T2- and T1-weighted images. Lim and colleagues [61] reported that 63% (27 of 43) of RF-ablated HCC showed air within the necrotic cavity on short-term follow-up examinations.

The probe track can often be identified after ablation as a linear defect extending from the liver surface into the interior of the necrotic cavity. On MR imaging, the track is characterized by low signal intensity on T2-weighted images, low signal on T1-weighted images, and lack of enhancement after contrast administration. An enhancing region of parenchyma surrounding the probe track may be observed because of edema and inflammation. Similarly, a small fluid collection may be present in the initial few weeks after procedure, along the liver surface at the entry site of the probe into the parenchyma.

Perfusion abnormalities may be present after ablative therapy because of parenchymal injury. Parenchymal injury may be caused by altered or obstructed vascular structures and generally disappear within 1 month of the intervention [61,66]. On MR images, perfusion abnormalities appear as wedge-shaped or patchy areas of enhancement on arterial-dominant phase images [67].

Within 6 to 12 months of ablation, the necrotic cavity may demonstrate considerable reduction in size (Fig. 2) [16]. Small necrotic cavities may result in focal hepatic atrophy with capsule retraction or disappear completely.

Liver transplantation

After surgery, both donors and recipients of living-related hemiliver donation are assessed for liver regeneration. The first evaluation of the liver volume should be performed 7 days after transplantation (baseline) and the following examination at the end of the first month (Fig. 3) [68].

Unsuccessful treatment

Liver resection

It is critically important to identify enhanced areas adjacent to the resected region because they may represent persistent or recurrent hypervascular malignant lesions, such as HCC or metastases [69]. Often, tumor recurrence has a similar appearance as untreated malignancy (ie, recurrences may be round or oval shaped with moderately high signal intensity on T2-weighted images and exhibit heterogeneous moderate or intense enhancement on arterial-dominant phase images). On portal and/or interstitial phase images, malignant focal liver lesions have a tendency to washout, a feature that is not seen in nonneoplastic areas.

Systemic chemotherapy

The increase in number, and size, and/or extent of enhancement on hepatic arterial-dominant phase

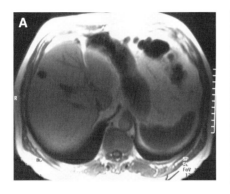
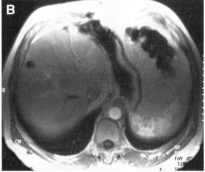
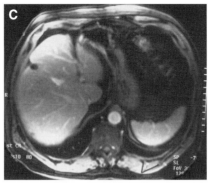

Fig. 2. Successful RF ablation. Transverse T1-weighted SGE (*A*), immediate postgadolinium SGE (*B*), and 90-second fat-suppressed postgadolinium SGE (*C*) images in a patient who underwent RF ablation months earlier. There is focus in the right hepatic lobe that shows low signal intensity and lack of enhancement (*A – C*). Note that the area has a smooth internal contour and there is adjacent liver retraction. These findings are consistent with successful response after RF ablation.

images of tumors after systemic chemotherapy is suggestive of nonresponse [54].

Transcatheter arterial chemoembolization

Any focally enhanced area after contrast administration within the necrotic cavity post–transcatheter arterial chemoembolization is consistent with residual or recurrent tumor [41,58].

Ablated lesions

Tumors that are incompletely ablated often demonstrate a nodule abutting the necrotic cavity and distorting the inner tumor margin [16,47,59,70]. The focus corresponds to the residual tumor and exhibits moderate high signal intensity on T2-weighted images and often enhances moderately or intensely on arterial-dominant phase images (Fig. 4). Tumors

with hypovascular characteristics before ablation (ie, metastasis from colon cancer) may have residual tumor with an appearance of late enhancement [17]. The depiction of residual tumor is facilitated by the contrast between the high signal nodule and the low signal background of the necrotic cavity on MR studies.

Although it is reported that residual tumors can be detected by imaging methods immediately after ablative therapy [16,61], they are more likely to be depicted at 1-month follow-up examinations [61,71]. Indeed, the variability in the signal intensity on T2- and T1-weighted images of the necrotic cavity during the first weeks after treatment may mask the presence of residual tumors [16]. Lim and colleagues [61] reported that 21% (8 of 38) of residual HCC had unremarkable 1-month follow-up CT but recurrent tumors were depicted at 4 to 13 months after ablation.

Other features that are highly suggestive of unsuccessful ablative therapy are the enlargement of the necrotic cavity within 1 month after the intervention

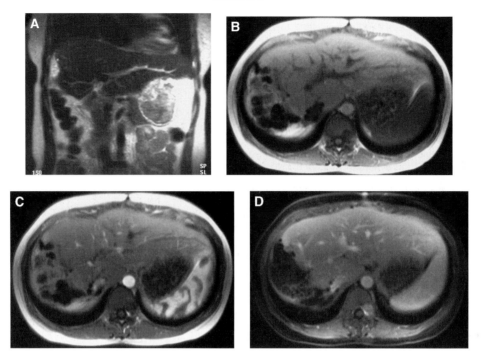

Fig. 3. Liver transplant. Coronal T2-weighted SS-ETSE (*A*), transverse SGE (*B*), immediate postgadolinium SGE (*C*), and 90-second fat-suppressed postgadolinium SGE (*D*) images in a patient who underwent liver transplantation. All vessels are patent. No perihepatic fluid collection or other complications are observed. Note the clips surrounding the inferior vena cava (*B*).

and the appearance of a thickened and irregular peripheral rim enhancement [60,72].

Post–liver transplant

In the transplanted liver, HCC may recur as metastatic lesions from the original tumor that was present in the explanted liver or, rarely, appear de novo. Recurrence occurs because of the spread of tumor cells by hematogenous, lymphatic, or peritoneal routes. De novo HCC are usually associated with immunosuppressive treatment [73,74].

CT or MR imaging for follow-up

Most studies have assessed the tumor response or treatment effectiveness by CT examination [19,22,34,70,72,75], because its low cost and the feasibility make this method very attractive to clinicians and radiologists. The superiority of MR imaging over CT with respect to the detection and characterization of focal liver lesions, however, is well known [29,30]. Although few studies compare the ability of CT and MR imaging regarding the detection of residual or recurrent tumors after treat-

ment, there is suggestive evidence that MR imaging is more accurate [21,47,54,71]. Dromain and colleagues [47] found MR imaging to be more sensitive and specific in the detection of residual or recurrent HCC after RF ablation. The authors suggested that the advantage of MR imaging over CT is achieved by T2-weighted images. The authors' experience suggests it is the greater enhancement appreciated on hepatic arterial-dominant phase images over analogous CT images supplemented with T2 information.

The early depiction of residual or recurrent tumor and recognition of treatment failure are important for planning new interventions. There is suggestive evidence that residual or recurrent tumors post–RF ablation acquire an irregular shape not easily assessed or treated in a new intervention [71].

Protocol for follow-up

Follow-up examinations after systemic chemotherapy are primarily performed to assess the patient's response and they are often at the discretion of the oncologist. The schedule of follow-up examination varies on a patient-by-patient basis and is commonly planned at the end of the treatment cycle.

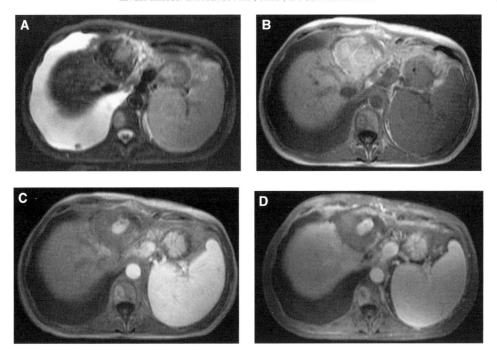

Fig. 4. Residual or recurrent tumor after RF ablation. Transverse T2-weighted SS-ETSE (*A*), T1-weighted SGE (*B*), immediate postgadolinium SGE (*C*), and 90-second fat-suppressed postgadolinium SGE (*D*) images in a patient who underwent RF ablation 6 months earlier. There is a round focus with irregular internal contour within the left hepatic lobe that demonstrates low signal intensity on T2-weighted image (*A*) and heterogeneous high signal intensity on T1-weighted image (*B*) compatible with an ablated area. Within this area, there is an oval lesion that shows high signal intensity on T2-weighted image (*A*), which enhances intensely on the early postgadolinium image (*C*) and remains enhanced on the late postgadolinium image (*D*). This area is compatible with tumor recurrence or residual tumor after RF ablation.

After ablative interventions, follow-up examinations are performed to evaluate the treatment effectiveness and the extent of potential complications. There is no consensus regarding the best timing for follow-up examinations [15]. Each institution follows its own rules and it is mostly based on professional experience and the patient's clinical condition. It has been suggested [16,60], however, that the first follow-up examination (baseline) should be performed within a week of the procedure primarily to detect complications or gross residual tumor that requires new intervention. The following examinations should be performed every 3 to 4 months for 1 year, and then every 6 months during the following years.

Complications

One of the major roles of postprocedural imaging is to recognize complications that may have resulted from treatment [76]. Complications postablative therapies can be classified as minor and major [77,78].

Most common minor complications include pain, skin burn, fever, nausea, dyspnea, subcutaneous and subcapsular hematoma, biloma and nonsurgical intraperitoneal bleeding, pleural effusion, and pneumothorax. The most common major complications are hepatic abscess requiring intervention, hepatic infarction, liver decompensation, injury to bile ducts, intraperitoneal hemorrhage requiring surgery or blood transfusion, hemothorax, perforation of bowel wall, neoplastic seeding, and death [11,18–20,25, 76,79–81].

After liver transplantation, both donors and recipients are assessed for surgical complications, such as fluid collections, stenoses of vessels or bile ducts, and transplant rejection. Fluid collections are commonly observed and include hematomas, seromas, bilomas, abscesses, and simple ascites (Fig. 5) [82]. Periportal signal abnormalities are frequently present in transplanted livers and may be consistent with dilated lymphatics secondary to impaired drainage after surgery; however, other causes, such as lymphocytic infiltration caused by rejection, must be considered [83]. Beyond the immediate transplant

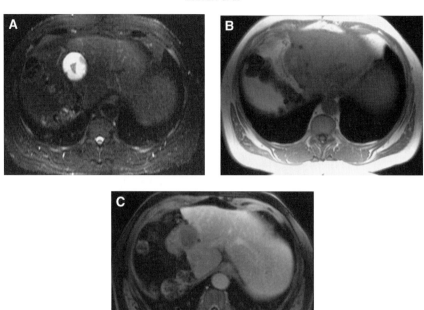

Fig. 5. Biloma after hemiliver donation. Transverse T2-weighted fat-suppressed SS-ETSE (*A*), T1-weighted SGE (*B*), and 90-second fat-suppressed postgadolinium SGE (*C*) images in a liver donor patient after resection. There is a rounded region located along the resection margin that exhibits high signal on the T2-weighted image (*A*), isointensity on the T1-weighted image (*B*), and faint perilesional enhancement on the late postgadolinium image (*C*) consistent with biloma.

period, expansion of the periportal tissue in a mass-like fashion may be an indication of posttransplant lymphoproliferative disorder [82]. Vascular complications, such as thrombosis and stenosis, are important causes of graft failure [84].

In the immediate postoperative period, up to 1 week or more, the current standard of practice is to use Doppler ultrasound to image for vascular complications, and CT to evaluate for tubes, catheters, drains, and other surgical devices to assess their appropriate locations. Later posttransplant imaging is probably better performed by MR imaging, which can also assess for tumor recurrence and late transplant complications.

Summary

Imaging investigation can assess the pretreatment, treatment-in-progress, and posttreatment liver. The higher diagnostic accuracy and greater patient safety of MR imaging may make it the modality-of-choice for these investigations. The previously described findings, however, may also be observed on CT and potentially also with contrast-enhanced ultrasound, and these findings should also be considered applicable to those modalities. Imaging guidance during interventional procedures is generally performed with ultrasound, as is assessment of liver in the immediate posttransplant setting.

References

[1] Bilimoria MM, Lauwers GY, Doherty DA, et al, International Cooperative Study Group on Hepatocellular Carcinoma. Underlying liver disease, not tumor factors, predicts long-term survival after resection of hepatocellular carcinoma. Arch Surg 2001;136:528–35.

[2] Harmon KE, Ryan Jr JA, Biehl TR, et al. Benefits and safety of hepatic resection for colorectal metastases. Am J Surg 1999;177:402–4.

[3] Holbrook RF, Koo K, Ryan JA. Resection of malignant primary liver tumors. Am J Surg 1996;171:453–5.

[4] Selzner M, Morse MA, Vredenburgh JJ, et al. Liver metastases from breast cancer: long-term survival after curative resection. Surgery 2000;127:383–9.

[5] Vlastos G, Smith DL, Singletary SE, et al. Long-term survival after an aggressive surgical approach in

patients with breast cancer hepatic metastases. Ann Surg Oncol 2004;11:869–74.

[6] Semelka RC, Worawattanakul S, Noone TC, et al. Chemotherapy-treated liver metastases mimicking hemangiomas on MR images. Abdom Imaging 1999; 24:378–82.

[7] Worawattanakul S, Semelka RC, Kelekis NL, et al. Angiosarcoma of the liver: MR imaging pre- and post-chemotherapy. Magn Reson Imaging 1997;15:613–7.

[8] Lang EK, Brown Jr CL. Colorectal metastases to the liver: selective chemoembolization. Radiology 1993; 189:417–22.

[9] Tellez C, Benson III AB, Lyster MT, et al. Phase II trial of chemoembolization for the treatment of metastatic colorectal carcinoma to the liver and review of the literature. Cancer 1998;82:1250–9.

[10] Ernst O, Sergent G, Mizrahi D, et al. Treatment of hepatocellular carcinoma by transcatheter arterial chemoembolization: comparison of planned periodic chemoembolization and chemoembolization based on tumor response. AJR Am J Roentgenol 1999;172: 59–64.

[11] Martinelli DJ, Wadler S, Bakal CW, et al. Utility of embolization or chemoembolization as second-line treatment in patients with advanced or recurrent colorectal carcinoma. Cancer 1994;74:1706–12.

[12] Ruszniewski P, Rougier P, Rcche A, et al. Hepatic arterial chemoembolization in patients with liver metastases of endocrine tumors: a prospective phase II study in 24 patients. Cancer 1993;71: 2624–30.

[13] Sakurai M, Okamura J, Kuroda C. Transcatheter chemo-embolization effective for treating hepatocellular carcinoma: a histopathologic study. Cancer 1984; 54:387–92.

[14] Yamada R, Sato M, Kawabata M, et al. Hepatic artery embolization in 120 patients with unresectable hepatoma. Radiology 1983;148:397–401.

[15] Goldberg SN, Gazelle GS, Compton CC, et al. Treatment of intrahepatic malignancy with radiofrequency ablation: radiologic-pathologic correlation. Cancer 2000;88:2452–63.

[16] Goldberg SN, Gazelle GS, Mueller PR. Thermal ablation therapy for focal malignancy: a unified approach to underlying principles, techniques, and diagnostic imaging guidance. AJR Am J Roentgenol 2000; 174:323–31.

[17] Goldberg SN, Charboneau JW, Dodd III GD, et al, International Working Group on Image-Guided Tumor Ablation. Image-guided tumor ablation: proposal for standardization of terms and reporting criteria. Radiology 2003;228:335–45.

[18] Lencioni RA, Allgaier HP, Cioni D, et al. Small hepatocellular carcinoma in cirrhosis: randomized comparison of radio-frequency thermal ablation versus percutaneous ethanol injection. Radiology 2003;228: 235–40.

[19] Livraghi T, Goldberg SN, Lazzaroni S, et al. Small hepatocellular carcinoma: treatment with radio-frequency ablation versus ethanol injection. Radiology 1999;210:655–61.

[20] Shibata T, Iimuro Y, Yamamoto Y, et al. Small hepatocellular carcinoma: comparison of radio-frequency ablation and percutaneous microwave coagulation therapy. Radiology 2002;223:331–7.

[21] de Baere T, Elias D, Dromain C, et al. Radiofrequency ablation of 100 hepatic metastases with a mean follow-up of more than 1 year. AJR Am J Roentgenol 2000; 175:1619–25.

[22] Pacella CM, Bizzarri G, Cecconi P, et al. Hepatocellular carcinoma: long-term results of combined treatment with laser thermal ablation and transcatheter arterial chemoembolization. Radiology 2001;219:669–78.

[23] Vogl TJ, Mack MG, Balzer JO, et al. Liver metastases: neoadjuvant downsizing with transarterial chemoembolization before laser-induced thermotherapy. Radiology 2003;229:457–64.

[24] Vogl TJ, Straub R, Eichler K, et al. Colorectal carcinoma metastases in liver: laser-induced interstitial thermotherapy–local tumor control rate and survival data. Radiology 2004;230:450–8.

[25] Mack MG, Straub R, Eichler K, et al. Breast cancer metastases in liver: laser-induced interstitial thermotherapy—local tumor control rate and survival data. Radiology 2004;233:400–9.

[26] Shankar S, Vansonnenberg E, Morrison PR, et al. Combined radiofrequency and alcohol injection for percutaneous hepatic tumor ablation. AJR Am J Roentgenol 2004;183:1425–9.

[27] Pichlmayr R, Weimann A, Tusch G, et al. Indications and role of liver transplantation for malignant tumors. Oncologist 1997;2:164–70.

[28] Rosado B, Gores GJ. Liver transplantation for neuroendocrine tumors: progress and uncertainty. Liver Transpl 2004;10:712–3.

[29] Semelka RC, Worawattanakul S, Kelekis NL, et al. Liver lesion detection, characterization, and effect on patient management: comparison of single-phase spiral CT and current MR techniques. J Magn Reson Imaging 1997;7:1040–7.

[30] Semelka RC, Martin DR, Balci C, et al. Focal liver lesions: comparison of dual-phase CT and multi-sequence multiplanar MR imaging including dynamic gadolinium enhancement. J Magn Reson Imaging 2001;13:397–401.

[31] Yamashita Y, Mitsuzaki K, Yi T, et al. Small hepatocellular carcinoma in patients with chronic liver damage: prospective comparison of detection with dynamic MR imaging and helical CT of the whole liver. Radiology 1996;200:79–84.

[32] Lencioni R, Cioni D, Crocetti L, et al. Percutaneous ablation of hepatocellular carcinoma: state-of-the-art. Liver Transpl 2004;10(2 Suppl 1):S91–7.

[33] Hasegawa S, Yamasaki N, Hiwaki T, et al. Factors that predict intrahepatic recurrence of hepatocellular carcinoma in 81 patients initially treated by percutaneous ethanol injection. Cancer 1999;86:1682–90.

[34] Livraghi T, Goldberg SN, Lazzaroni S, et al. Hepato-

cellular carcinoma: radio-frequency ablation of medium and large lesions. Radiology 2000;214:761–8.

[35] Dodd III GD, Soulen MC, Kane RA, et al. Minimally invasive treatment of malignant hepatic tumors: at the threshold of a major breakthrough. Radiographics 2000;20:9–27.

[36] Kitamoto M, Imagawa M, Yamada H, et al. Radio-frequency ablation in the treatment of small hepatocellular carcinomas: comparison of the radiofrequency effect with and without chemoembolization. AJR Am J Roentgenol 2003;181:997–1003.

[37] Couinaud C. Le foie: etudes anatomiques et chirurgicales. Paris: Masson; 1957.

[38] McGhana JP, Dodd III GD. Radiofrequency ablation of the liver: current status. AJR Am J Roentgenol 2001;176:3–16.

[39] Goldberg SN, Hahn PF, Halpern EF, et al. Radiofrequency tissue ablation: effect of pharmacologic modulation of blood flow on coagulation diameter. Radiology 1998;209:761–7.

[40] Semelka RC, Braga L, Armao D, et al. Liver. In: Semelka RC, editor. Abdominal-pelvic MRI. New York: Wiley-Liss; 2002. p. 33–317.

[41] Semelka RC, Worawattanakul S, Mauro MA, et al. Malignant hepatic tumors: changes on MRI after hepatic arterial chemoembolization—preliminary findings. J Magn Reson Imaging 1998;8:48–56.

[42] Matsumoto R, Oshio K, Jolesz FA. Monitoring of laser and freezing-induced ablation in the liver with T1-weighted MR imaging. J Magn Reson Imaging 1992; 2:555–62.

[43] Vogl TJ, Muller PK, Hammerstingl R, et al. Malignant liver tumors treated with MR imaging-guided laser-induced thermotherapy: technique and prospective results. Radiology 1995;196:257–65.

[44] Libshitz HI, Jing BS, Wallace S, et al. Sterilized metastases: a diagnostic and therapeutic dilemma. AJR Am J Roentgenol 1983;140:15–9.

[45] Jeong YY, Mitchell DG, Hann HW, et al. Hepatocellular carcinoma after systemic chemotherapy: gadolinium-enhanced MR measurement of necrosis by volume histogram. Comput Assist Tomogr 2001;25:624–8.

[46] Takashimizu I, Ohkusa T, Okayasu I, et al. Comparison of necrosis and fibrotic repair after ethanol injection between normal and cirrhotic livers. Digestion 1997; 58:384–8.

[47] Dromain C, de Baere T, Elias D, et al. Hepatic tumors treated with percutaneous radio-frequency ablation: CT and MR imaging follow-up. Radiology 2002;223: 255–62.

[48] Ebara M, Kita K, Sugiura N, et al. Therapeutic effect of percutaneous ethanol injection on small hepatocellular carcinoma: evaluation with CT. Radiology 1995; 195:371–7.

[49] Goshima S, Kanematsu M, Matsuo M, et al. Early-enhancing nonneoplastic lesions on gadolinium-enhanced magnetic resonance imaging of the liver following partial hepatectomy. J Magn Reson Imaging 2004;20:66–74.

[50] Arrive L, Hricak H, Goldberg HI, et al. MR appearance of the liver after partial hepatectomy. AJR Am J Roentgenol 1989;152:1215–20.

[51] Haran EF, Maretzek AF, Goldberg I, et al. Tamoxifen enhances cell death in implanted MCF7 breast cancer by inhibiting endothelium growth. Cancer Res 1994; 54:5511–4.

[52] Ohtomo K, Itai Y, Yoshikawa K, et al. MR imaging of hepatoma treated by embolization. J Comput Assist Tomogr 1986;10:973–5.

[53] De Santis M, Torricelli P, Christani A, et al. MRI of hepatocellular carcinoma before and after transcatheter chemoembolization. J Comput Assist Tomogr 1993; 17:901–8.

[54] Braga L, Semelka RC, Pietrobon R, et al. Does hypervascularity of liver metastases as detected on MRI predict disease progression in breast cancer patients? AJR Am J Roentgenol 2004;182:1207–13.

[55] Semelka RC. Metastatic liver tumor: circumferential versus wedge-shaped perilesional enhancement and quantitative image and pathologic correlation. Radiology 2001;219:298–300.

[56] Semelka RC, Hussain SM, Marcos HB, et al. Perilesional enhancement of hepatic metastases: correlation between MR imaging and histphatologic findings: initial observations. Radiology 2000;215:89–94.

[57] Arisawa Y, Sutanto-Ward E, Fortunato L, et al. Hepatic artery dexamethasone infusion inhibits colorectal hepatic metastases: a regional antiangiogenesis therapy. Ann Surg Oncol 1995;2:114–20.

[58] Bartolozzi C, Lencioni R, Caramella D, et al. Hepatocellular carcinoma: CT and MR features after transcatheter arterial embolization and percutaneous ethanol injection. Radiology 1994;191:123–8.

[59] Kuszyk BS, Boitnott JK, Choti MA, et al. Local tumor recurrence following hepatic cryoablation: radiologic-histopathologic correlation in a rabbit model. Radiology 2000;217:477–86.

[60] Limanond P, Zimmerman P, Raman SS, et al. Interpretation of CT and MRI after radiofrequency ablation of hepatic malignancies. AJR Am J Roentgenol 2003;181:1635–40.

[61] Lim HK, Choi D, Lee WJ, et al. Hepatocellular carcinoma treated with percutaneous radio-frequency ablation: evaluation with follow-up multiphase helical CT. Radiology 2001;221:447–54.

[62] Cotran RS, Kumar V, Collins T. Robbins' pathologic basis of disease. 6th edition. Philadelphia: Saunders; 1999.

[63] Rubin E, Farber JL. Pathology. 3rd edition. Philadelphia: Lippincott-Raven; 1999.

[64] Joseph FB, Baumgarten DA, Bernardino ME. Hepatocellular carcinoma: CT appearance after percutaneous ethanol ablation therapy. Work in progress. Radiology 1993;186:553–6.

[65] Mitsuzaki K, Yamashita Y, Nishiharu T, et al. CT appearance of hepatic tumors after microwave coagulation therapy. AJR Am J Roentgenol 1998;171: 1397–403.

[66] Schlund JF, Semelka RC, Kettritz U, et al. Correlation of perfusion abnormalities on CTAP and immediate postintravenous gadolinium-enhanced gradient echo MRI. Abdom Imaging 1996;21:49–52.

[67] Lencioni R, Cioni D, Bartolozzi C. Percutaneous radiofrequency thermal ablation of liver malignancies: techniques, indications, imaging findings, and clinical results. Abdom Imaging 2001;26:345–60.

[68] Bassignani MJ, Fulcher AS, Szucs RA, et al. Use of imaging for living donor liver transplantation. Radiographics 2001;21:39–52.

[69] Soyer P, Bluemke DA, Zeitoun G, et al. Detection of recurrent hepatic metastases after partial hepatectomy: value of CT combined with arterial portography. AJR Am J Roentgenol 1994;162:1327–30.

[70] Chopra S, Dodd III GD, Chanin MP, et al. Radiofrequency ablation of hepatic tumors adjacent to the gallbladder: feasibility and safety. AJR Am J Roentgenol 2003;180:697–701.

[71] Gazelle GS, Goldberg SN, Solbiati L, et al. Tumor ablation with radio-frequency energy. Radiology 2000; 217:633–46.

[72] Choi D, Lim HK, Kim MJ, et al. Recurrent hepatocellular carcinoma: percutaneous radiofrequency ablation after hepatectomy. Radiology 2004;230:135–41.

[73] Flemming P, Tillmann HL, Barg-Hock H, et al. Donor origin of de novo hepatocellular carcinoma in hepatic allografts. Transplantation 2003;76:871–3.

[74] Schlitt HJ, Neipp M, Weimann A, et al. Recurrence patterns of hepatocellular and fibrolamellar carcinoma after liver transplantation. Clin Oncol 1999;17:324–31.

[75] Pacella CM, Bizzarri G, Magnolfi F, et al. Laser thermal ablation in the treatment of small hepatocellular carcinoma: results in 74 patients. Radiology 2001;221:712–20.

[76] Rhim H, Yoon KH, Lee JM, et al. Major complications after radio-frequency thermal ablation of hepatic tumors: spectrum of imaging findings. Radiographics 2003;23:123–34.

[77] Burke DR, Lewis CA, Cardella JF, et al. Quality improvement guidelines for percutaneous transhepatic cholangiography and biliary drainage. Society of Cardiovascular and Interventional Radiology. J Vasc Interv Radiol 1997;8:677–81.

[78] Lewis CA, Allen TE, Burke DR, et al. Quality improvement guidelines for central venous access. The Standards of Practice Committee of the Society of Cardiovascular & Interventional Radiology. J Vasc Interv Radiol 1997;8:475–9.

[79] de Baere T, Risse O, Kuoch V, et al. Adverse events during radiofrequency treatment of 582 hepatic tumors. AJR Am J Roentgenol 2003;181:695–700.

[80] Rhim H, Dodd III GD, Chintapalli KN, et al. Radiofrequency thermal ablation of abdominal tumors: lessons learned from complications. Radiographics 2004;24:41–52.

[81] Vogl TJ, Straub R, Eichler K, et al. Malignant liver tumors treated with MR imaging-guided laser-induced thermotherapy: experience with complications in 899 patients (2,520 lesions). Radiology 2002;225:367–77.

[82] Ito K, Siegelman ES, Stolpen AH, et al. MR imaging of complications after liver transplantation. AJR Am J Roentgenol 2000;175:1145–9.

[83] Marincek B, Barbier PA, Becker CD, et al. CT appearance of impaired lymphatic drainage in liver transplants. AJR Am J Roentgenol 1986;147:519–23.

[84] Glockner JF, Forauer AR, Solomon H, et al. Three-dimensional gadolinium-enhanced MR angiography of vascular complications after liver transplantation. AJR Am J Roentgenol 2000;174:1447–53.

RADIOLOGIC
CLINICS
of North America

Radiol Clin N Am 43 (2005) 929 – 947

Hepatic Imaging: Comparison of Modalities

Shahid M. Hussain, MD[a],*, Richard C. Semelka, MD[b]

[a]Section of Abdominal Imaging, Department of Radiology, Erasmus MC, Dr. Molewaterplein 40,
3015 GD Rotterdam, The Netherlands
[b]Department of Radiology, School of Medicine, University of North Carolina at Chapel Hill, Chapel Hill, NC, USA

Focal and diffuse liver abnormalities are common disease processes. In particular, it should be recognized that benign focal liver lesions, including cysts, hemangiomas, biliary hamartomas, and focal nodular hyperplasia, are common. The exact prevalence of benign liver masses is unknown, but some studies suggest that these lesions may be found in more than 20% of the general population [1]. Recent studies suggest that small (<15 mm) liver lesions seen at CT are benign in more than 80% of patients with known malignancy [2]. With the use of multirow detector CT and thinner collimation, it is likely that more liver lesions will be detected that need additional imaging for characterization [3–5]. The most common malignant liver lesions are metastases. Most of these originate from colorectal malignancies. The most common primary malignant liver lesions include hepatocellular carcinomas (HCC) and intrahepatic cholangiocarcinoma. In addition, the liver is commonly involved in (1) diffuse (parenchymal and depositional) diseases including steatosis, hemochromatosis, hepatitis, fibrosis, and cirrhosis; (2) biliary tree abnormalities including stone disease, Caroli's disease, primary sclerosing cholangitis, and extrahepatic or hilar cholangiocarcinoma; and (3) vascular abnormalities including portal hypertension, portal vein thrombosis, arterioportal shunts, and Budd-Chiari syndrome.

A primary objective in imaging the liver is to distinguish benign from metastatic and primary malignant lesions. Several malignancies, such as breast, pancreas, and colorectal tumors, have a particular propensity to metastasize to the liver. Colorectal liver metastases are the most common of these. In the United States, more than 50% of patients (in 1998, 56,000 of 131,600 patients) who die from colorectal cancer have liver metastases at autopsy [6]. Of those who have colorectal liver metastases, 10% to 25% are candidates for surgical resection, and the 5-year survival rate following resection of isolated colorectal liver metastases can be as high as 38% [6]. Without any treatment, the survival rate is less than 1% [6]. For the remaining 75% to 90% of patients with liver metastases who are not amenable to surgery, several new therapies have been developed [6].

Generally, 1% to 2% of patients with cirrhosis develop HCC. The 5-year survival rate of patients with HCC with treatment can be as high as 75%, and without treatment less than 5% [7]. It is important to recognize that a hypervascular liver lesion in the setting of cirrhosis has a relatively narrow differential diagnosis, including HCC; high-grade dysplastic nodule; small hemangioma; and focal early enhancing tissue (often small foci of acute-on-chronic inflammation or vascular anomaly). A hypervascular liver lesion in a noncirrhotic liver has a much wider differential diagnosis including HCC in a noncirrhotic liver, hepatocellular adenoma, focal nodular hyperplasia, hypervascular metastases, small hemangiomas, and vascular shunts. It should be noted that HCC in a noncirrhotic liver is not rare [8].

* Corresponding author.
  E-mail address: s.hussain@erasmusmc.nl
(S.M. Hussain).

This article describes a number of aspects of liver imaging, including the main reasons for imaging of the liver; the current status and the recent developments of ultrasound (US), CT, MR imaging, and PET; and the role of these imaging modalities in the assessment of hepatic abnormalities. Finally, a systematic review of the current relevant literature on studies that compare modalities is presented, and a strategy for the work-up of the liver diseases is proposed.

Imaging of the liver

Annually, thousands of patients worldwide undergo imaging for the work-up of a suspected or known abnormality of the liver. Cross-sectional imaging modalities, such as US, CT, and MR imaging, are used in most centers to assess liver abnormalities. These modalities, often used in various combinations, have fundamental differences in data acquisition and hence differences in the type of physical characteristics of tissues that they interrogate (Table 1).

Aspects of the identified liver abnormalities influence the clinical and surgical decision making: (1) benign abnormalities, such as cysts, biliary hamartomas [9], and hemangiomas [10,11], do not require treatment and often minimal follow-up; (2) benign abnormalities, such as focal nodular hyperplasia and hepatocellular adenomas, may require treatment in some cases [12]; (3) malignant lesions that originate from the liver, such as HCC, often need liver transplantation or other forms of treatment; (4) metastatic liver lesions may or may not be amenable to resection or other forms of treatment [5,6,13,14]; (5) diffuse parenchymal abnormalities need initial assessment, follow-up, or monitoring of treatment; and (6) biliary

tree abnormalities require initial assessment, follow-up, or monitoring of treatment.

The main goals of imaging are to assess (1) the number and size of the liver abnormalities; (2) the location of abnormalities relative to the liver vessels; (3) the nature of the lesions (benign versus malignant); (4) the origin (primary versus secondary) of abnormalities; and (5) the liver parenchyma surrounding the lesions [6]. It is important to emphasize that distinction of benign from malignant lesions is critical.

Currently, there is no consensus concerning the optimal strategy for imaging the liver. Imaging modalities are often used based on the requests of referring physicians and the availability of equipment and experience of the radiologists. Most centers use US, CT, and US-guided biopsy. MR imaging is often used as a problem-solving modality. In addition, other modalities, such as CT arterioportography (CTAP), CT hepatic arteriography (CTHA), PET, and laparoscopy with or without intraoperative US, are also used depending on the availability and experience of the clinicians and radiologists.

Ultrasound

Because of the high incidence of benign liver abnormalities, such as cysts, hemangiomas, biliary hamartomas, and focal nodular hyperplasia, in the general population, the initial US for many patients is not the end but a beginning of an extensive and lengthy work-up. A typical example that is often encountered in the daily clinical routine is a relatively young female patient who undergoes an US of the upper abdomen, in whom a liver lesion is seen, which

Table 1
Comparison of the main imaging features of ultrasound, CT, and MR imaging

US	CT	MR imaging
Echogenecity differences	X-ray attenuation differences	Tissue relaxation time differences T1 and T2
Differential enhancement[a]	Differential enhancement (iodine)	Differential enhancement (gadolinium)
Doppler	—	Inflow (MRA)
Duplex	—	Phase contrast (MRA)
Image optimization techniques	—	Tissue specific contrast media
—	—	Chemical shift imaging
—	—	Selective tissue suppression and excitation
—	—	Fluid imaging (MRCP)
—	—	Diffusion imaging
—	—	MR spectroscopy
—	—	Nonproton metabolic imaging

Abbreviation: MRCP, MR cholangiopancreatography.

[a] The use of ultrasound contrast media with or without harmonic imaging is limited to a few centers worldwide.

needs further characterization [15]. After this initial US, the work-up can develop into many directions. US may be followed by a CT or an US-guided biopsy, or an MR imaging.

US is widely available, and many clinicians request US as the initial imaging modality for the assessment of the upper abdomen including the liver. In such cases, often there is a wide variety of indications including vague upper abdominal complaints, pain, or unexpected abnormal liver function tests. The aims of this strategy are to get additional information and to narrow down the differential diagnosis in what they hope is a relatively quick and cost-effective manner. Currently, US can be performed with good image quality. A number of technical developments are important to mention that have improved the image quality and diagnostic information of US in real time.

Tissue harmonics

Tissue harmonics is a signal processing function that changes the fundamental beam through either receiver filters or pulse inversion techniques. This results in the use of only the returning harmonic signal. The use of tissue harmonic function is possible in real time and can reduce haze, clutter, and image artifacts. Dramatic reduction in artifacts can be achieved in anechoic structures, such as vessels and cysts.

Contrast harmonics

Contrast harmonic imaging uses the harmonic properties and motion characteristics of microbubbles to display the contrast agents. When microbubbles are isonated, they reflect both fundamental and harmonic frequencies. By programming the US system to receive only the harmonic signals, the contrast agent can be visualized better and the echo signals from the surrounding tissue can be suppressed [16]. Most vendors apply pulsed inversion harmonics for contrast-enhanced US. For a detailed description and its application, please see the article by Kono and colleagues elsewhere in this issue.

Real-time spatial compound imaging

Real-time spatial compound imaging (SonoCT, Philips Medical Systems, Best, The Netherlands) is an ultrasound technique that uses electronic beam steering of a transducer array to acquire several (three to nine) overlapping images of an object from different view angles rapidly (Fig. 1). These single-angle scans are averaged to form a new multiangle compound image that is updated in real time with each subsequent scan. Compound imaging shows improved image quality compared with conventional US primarily because of reduction of speckle, clutter, and other acoustic artifacts [17].

Adaptive real-time image processing

This can continually provide image enhancement down to the pixel level.

Miscellaneous

These include automatic adjustment of the time gain compensation; panoramic imaging (expanded field of view); real-time three-dimensional and real-time multiplanar imaging; and improved color and power Doppler and duplex imaging. Most of these measures result in better image quality in real time (Fig. 2). These developments have consolidated the role of US in the current clinical practice. For hepatic imaging, the fundamental limitations of US remain. These include operator-dependency with low repro-

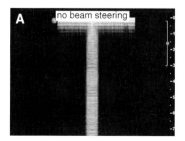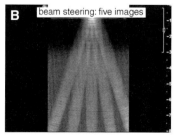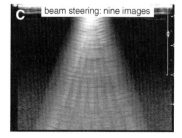

Fig. 1. Demonstration of real-time spatial compound imaging. A metal wire (a part of an opened paperclip) was imaged (7.5-MHz transducer) without electronic beam steering (*A*), beam steering with five overlapping images (*B*), and nine overlapping images (*C*). Eventually, the real-time spatial compound imaging (SonoCT, Philips Medical Systems, Best, The Netherlands) presents the data as a single image and updates this image in real-time.

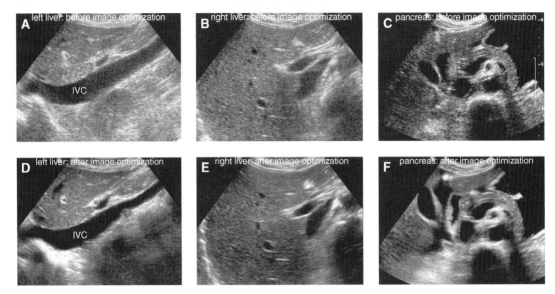

Fig. 2. Gray-scale US (image optimization). (A–C) US of the liver and pancreas before optimization. The images are course and grainy because of the presence of clutter and scatter artifacts. (D–F) US of the liver and pancreas after optimization. The images have better quality and appear sharper with more contrast, more anatomic detail, and less artifacts. This improvement in image quality was achieved in real-time (during scanning) with the use of real-time spatial compound imaging (SonoCT), automatic adjustment of time gain compensation, continuous real-time image enhancement at the pixel level (XRES), and tissue harmonics.

ducibility, lack of overview of the anatomy, and lack of technical ability to change the intrinsic tissue contrast (see Table 1). Contrast agents facilitate the characterization of a solitary known lesion, but do not allow surveying of the entire liver, which is virtually always an important aspect of a liver study. Multiple lesions may be present, including multiple lesions of different benign and malignant histologies. These limitations result in low sensitivity and specificity of US for liver abnormalities. In many centers, the clinical and surgical decision making does not take place based on the US of the liver alone.

CT

The broad availability of CT and the recent development and implementation of the faster multi-row detector machines make this modality an excellent tool for detection and characterization of focal liver lesions. Current CT scanners can obtain simultaneous multiple acquisitions per each gantry rotation. With the current multidetector CT, fast data acquisition over a large anatomic area (entire body with isometric voxels) is possible in less than 30 seconds. The isometric nature of the data facilitates high-quality reconstructions of mainly the vas-

cular and bony structures in any desirable anatomic orientation (Fig. 3).

The development of CT machines with multiple acquisitions per rotation capability began in 1992. Since then, the following progressive developments have occurred in CT technique:

1. 1992: dual-slice CT scanners
2. 1998: four-slice multidetector row scanners
3. 2001 and 2002: 8- to 16-detector row scanners
4. 2003: 32- to 64-detector row scanners;
5. 2003: the rotation speed of the gantry decreased to 0.33 seconds

These technical developments of multidetector CT allow imaging of the entire liver in more than one pass in a single breathhold. The reduced temporal resolution of about 5 seconds for the whole liver allows perfusion studies of the liver. The shorter scan times also allow the capture of distinct phases, including the unenhanced phase, the arterial phase, the portal phase, and the venous phase. These phases provide important information concerning the enhancement patterns and hence the possibility of characterization of focal liver lesions. In clinical practice, however, the number of phases that are usually acquired with CT are limited and often kept to a minimum, mainly because of concerns about

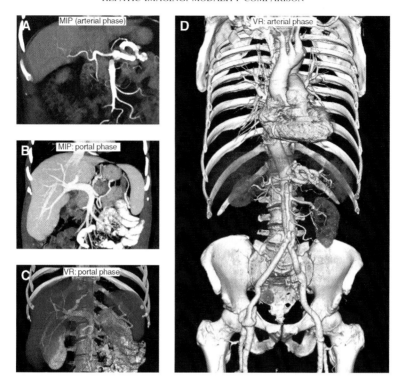

Fig. 3. A 16-slice CT examination of the chest and abdomen in the arterial and portal-venous phases (scan time 15 second per phase). (*A*) Coronal maximum-intensity projection (MIP) from the arterial phase shows the mesenteric and hepatic vessels. (*B*) Coronal MIP from the portal phase shows the portal vein. (*C*) Volume rendering (VR) based on the portal phase shows the relationship between vessels and organs. (*D*) The isometric nature of the voxels facilitates high-quality (almost anatomic) of the VR of the entire chest and abdomen.

radiation hazard. The issue of radiation is even more important in relatively young and otherwise healthy patients with an incidental liver lesion that needs characterization or follow-up.

One fundamental limitation of CT remains the lack of the ability to alter the intrinsic soft tissue contrast, which is useful to assess diffuse and focal liver abnormalities. At CT, evaluation of liver abnormalities is based on two basic parameters: attenuation differences and differential enhancement (see Table 1). The major achievement of multidetector CT is the large anatomic coverage (overall topographic display) and the superb imaging of the vascular anatomy and vascular abnormalities. A more detailed description of multidetector CT is presented by Aytekin and colleagues elsewhere in this issue.

PET

PET is an imaging modality that uses positron emitters, such as fluorine-18, to visualize tissues,

such as cancers with increased glucose metabolism. The most commonly used radiotracer for PET is 2-[^{18}F] fluoro-2-deoxy-D-glucose (FDG). FDG, like glucose, is taken up by cancer cells. In normal cells, glucose-6-phospate or FDG-6-phosphate can be dephosphorylated and exit the cells. In many cancer cells, however, expression of glucose-6-phosphatase is often significantly decreased; FDG-6-phosphate cannot be metabolized and is trapped in the cancer cells, and can be visualized by PET.

FDG-PET has been proved to be highly sensitive in detecting hepatic metastases from various primaries, such as colon, pancreas, esophagus, sarcoma, and parotid. Additionally, in the case of suspected recurrent colorectal cancer, FDG-PET may be more sensitive than CT for discovering hepatic metastases, with the potential of detecting disease earlier than CT, so that metastatic disease is more amenable to curative resection. FDG-PET should be considered in the setting of increasing serum carcinoembryonic antigen level to assess for hepatic metastases, because it has been shown to be more sensitive than CT for this purpose [18].

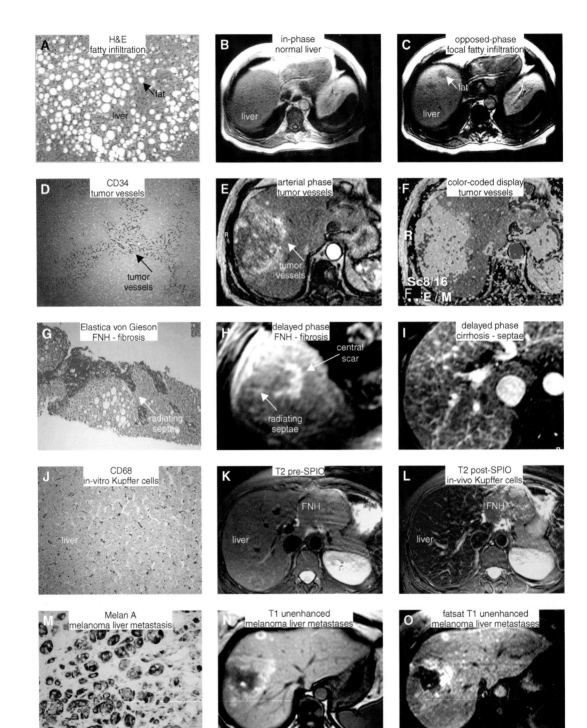

FDG-PET imaging has an important role in determining if there are (colorectal) metastases to the liver and whether disease has spread beyond the liver. Such information is critical for planning surgical resections of liver metastases. The sensitivity of FDG-PET for HCC is about 50%. Although FDG-PET can fail to detect many HCCs and their extrahepatic metastases, it does detect many of the poorly differentiated HCC. For benign primary liver lesions, like hemangioma, hepatocellular adenomas, and focal nodular hyperplasia, FDG-PET is also not suitable. Other PET tracers are being developed that improve the detection of primary liver lesions, such as HCC. Small-volume cholangiocarcinoma may also escape detection by FDG-PET; however, gallbladder carcinoma is generally well detected by FDG-PET. The ability of FDG-PET quantitatively to estimate metabolic rates makes it a potentially valuable tool for monitoring response to therapy, which will likely assume an expanding role for this modality.

False-negative FDG-PET has been reported caused by (1) lack of substantial uptake of FDG by malignant lesions; (2) underestimation of uptake; (3) mislocalization of foci; (4) recent completion of chemotherapy; (5) low spatial resolution; and (6) physiologic movement (eg, respiration) during emission scan, which is acquired during free breathing over several minutes. False-positive findings for malignancy on PET have also been reported caused by (1) intrahepatic abscess; (2) penetrating gallbladder empyema; and (3) benign inflammatory lesions, such as regenerative nodules in a cirrhotic liver.

In the near future, the detection of subcentimeter lesions will improve with the use of PET-CT, sophisticated image correction and reconstruction algorithms, and higher spatial resolution. For more detailed description of PET and its applications, the reader is directed to the article by Khandani and colleagues elsewhere in this issue.

MR imaging

MR imaging can provide comprehensive and highly accurate diagnostic information concerning diffuse (parenchymal or depositional) abnormalities, vascular and biliary anatomy and abnormalities, and focal liver abnormalities, obviating the need for other imaging modalities. Until recently, MR imaging has been used as a problem-solving modality because of the expense of the procedure. With increasing availability, MR imaging may be used as a first-line imaging modality with similar or greater accuracy, enabling a faster diagnostic and decision-making process that ultimately should prove more cost-effective.

Because of the unique ability of MR imaging to vary the intrinsic soft tissue characteristics and through the use of nonspecific and specific contrast media, MR imaging has become a versatile imaging modality. MR imaging can visualize several tissues and anatomic components of the liver separately based on T1-weighted imaging (including chemical shift imaging for the detection of small amounts of fat; fat-suppressed sequences for melanin and hemorrhage); T2-weighted imaging (distinction between solid and nonsolid liver lesions based on fluid content; MR cholangiopancreatography); diffusion-weighted imaging (lesion detection and characterization; black-blood imaging) [19]; flow-sensitive sequences (inflow MR angiography [MRA]; phase-contrast MRA); nonspecific contrast media (dynamic gadolinium-enhanced imaging for lesion detection and characterization; tumor vascularity background liver vascularity; contrast-enhanced MRA) [11,20]; and specific contrast media (distinction between primary and secondary liver lesions) [21–24]. These imaging properties allow highly detailed evaluation of diffuse and focal liver abnormalities. Because of the detailed, comprehensive information, current state-of-the-art MR imaging of the liver has parallels

Fig. 4. Hepatic MR imaging and its parallels with pathology. (A–C) Fatty infiltration. Before the era of MR imaging, pathology (hematoxylin and eosin stain) was the only method to detect fatty infiltration of the liver with certainty. Currently, chemical shift imaging (in-phase and opposed-phase) can readily detect fatty infiltration in vivo. (D–F) Tumor vessels. CD34 is a specific stain that can be used to demonstrate the presence of vessels in tumors. With gadolinium-enhanced MR imaging in the arterial phase, with or without pixel-wise color-coding, the tumor vessels can be visualized in vivo. Tumor vessels may also be detected using blood pool MR contrast media. (G–I) Fibrosis. Elastica von Gieson is a specific stain that can be used to demonstrate the presence of fibrosis and fibrotic septae, which can be used with focal nodular hyperplasia (FNH). With gadolinium-enhanced MR imaging in the delayed phase, the presence of fibrotic septae and central scar composed of fibrosis can be demonstrated accurately as areas of delayed progressive enhancement. (J–L) Kupffer cells. CD68 is a specific stain that can be used to demonstrate the presence of Kupffer cells in normal liver tissue and tumors of hepatocellular origin in vitro. Superparamagnetic iron-oxide MR imaging contrast media lower the signal intensity of tissues containing Kupffer cells because of uptake of contrast in these cells, which can be used in vivo to demonstrate the hepatocellular origin of tumors and tissues (eg, FNH and normal liver). (M–O) Melanin. Melan A is a specific stain that can be used to demonstrate the presence of melanin in tissue and tumors in vitro (melanoma and its metastases). Unenhanced T1-weighted MR imaging with or without frequency-selective fat-suppression can demonstrate melanin-containing melanoma metastases confidently in vivo.

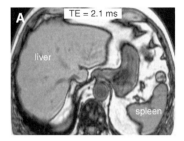 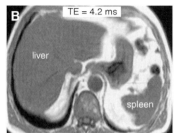 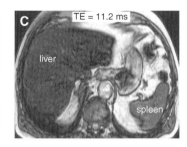

Fig. 5. Iron deposition in the liver and spleen. Increasing TE values of 2.1 milliseconds (*A*), 4.2 milliseconds (*B*), and 11.2 milliseconds (*C*) show progressive decrease in the signal intensity of the liver and spleen because of iron deposition within Kupffer cells.

with pathology (Fig. 4). This facilitates evaluation and follow-up after treatment of diffuse depositional liver disease in a noninvasive manner (Fig. 5), and posttherapy changes in malignant hepatic lesions.

Recent emerging developments have occurred in MR imaging that are important for body MR imaging applications. These include (1) recent technical developments, (2) parallel MR imaging, and (3) development of 3-T whole-body MR systems. The following developments are important to emphasize:

1. Increased main magnetic field strength with resultant higher signal-to-noise ratio.
2. Improved radiofrequency coil design (from large single-body or a single-surface coil to arrays of multiple smaller (phased-array) coils, currently containing 4 to 8 elements, and 16 to 32 elements or higher in the near future).
3. Improved bandwidth per receiver channel (3 MHz) with advances in digital electronics for faster readouts and faster reconstructions of k-space data sets.
4. Increased gradient performance (from gradients of < 10 mT/m with switching rates of > 1 milliseconds to gradients with >50 mT/m with switching rates in the order of 100 microseconds; these gradients can achieve lower TR and TE values and allow better spatial and temporal coverage and drastically reduce dead time periods during which no MR signal is acquired.
5. Newer and faster acquisition methods and sequences, such as various forms of echo train and echo planar T2-weighted and T1-weighted three-dimensional gradient-echo sequences.
6. Parallel MR imaging: the basis of this technique is the use of multiple independent receiver coils with distinct sensitivities across the object being imaged. In conventional MR imaging, the role of phased-array coils was merely

to improve signal-to-noise ratio, whereas in parallel imaging the phased-array coils are used to reduce the scan time. Application of parallel imaging includes (1) higher temporal resolution (faster imaging; eg, MR imaging exams in non-cooperative patients, time-resolved MRA, and perfusion studies); (2) higher spatial resolution (larger matrices, thinner slices [eg, high-resolution MRA]); (3) reduced effective interecho spacing (less image blurring and image distortion in echo-train spin echo and echo planar imaging [eg, high-quality MR cholangiopancreatography and single-shot echo planar imaging of the abdomen]); and (4) reduced specific absorption rate caused by shorter echo-trains (important for optimization of body MR imaging sequences at 3 T).
7. MR imaging at 3 T: currently, the greatest advantage of the higher signal-to-noise ratio of 3 T in body imaging, using a combination of eight-channel torso phased-array coils, higher (>2) acceleration factors, and gadolinium enhancement, is the use of three-dimensional gradient echo gadolinium-enhanced sequences for the liver. This allows higher in-plane and through-plane spatial resolution. Considerable sequence optimization remains to be done at 3 T. A more detailed description of the role of MR imaging in the assessment of liver lesions appears in the article by Martin and colleagues elsewhere in this issue.

Role of various modalities for hepatic imaging

Focal liver lesions

Primarily reflecting the increased use of cross-sectional imaging modalities and the high prevalence of benign liver lesions, incidental detection of liver

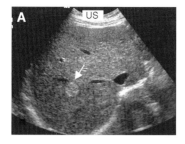 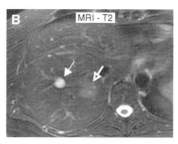 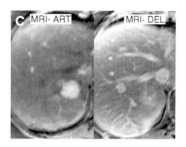

Fig. 6. Hemangioma and FNH: US versus MR imaging. (*A*) US of the liver shows an echogenic lesion (*arrow*) in segment VII of the liver. MR imaging was performed for further characterization. (*B*) T2-weighted image showed two lesions: one was much brighter than the liver (*solid arrow*) and the second slightly higher signal than the liver (*open arrow*). (*C*) Gadolinium-enhanced MR imaging in the arterial phase shows intense homogenous enhancement of the larger lesion, whereas the smaller one shows peripheral nodular enhancement. In the delayed phase (*C*), the larger lesion becomes almost isointense with enhancement of a small central scar, whereas the smaller lesion retains contrast. The MR imaging findings were typical for a hemangioma (small lesion) and an FNH.

lesions is common. In such cases, US is regularly the initial examination. Cysts and cystic liver lesions, including dilated bile ducts, are easier to detect than solid liver lesions at US. At US, color Doppler can be used in real-time to assess the vascular versus nonvascular nature of liver lesions. Noncystic liver lesions in an otherwise normal liver may have similar echogenicity to each other and to the background liver, and may be difficult to detect and characterize at US (Fig. 6). Most centers do not routinely use US contrast media for improved detection and characterization, in part because many are not approved for use at present, and mainly because most centers use CT or MR imaging in this capacity to form medical and surgical decision making. CT and MR imaging provide reproducible image quality with better anatomic detail and topographic display, which is essential information for planning surgery or other

procedures. A biopsy is often unnecessary if the liver lesion has a classical appearance on CT or MR imaging (Fig. 7).

The fundamental limitation of CT is its lack of intrinsic soft tissue contrast and its moderate sensitivity for the presence of intravenous contrast. For detection and characterization, CT mainly relies on high in-plane spatial resolution and vascularity of liver lesions. Small liver lesions (<2 cm), which are now more often detected on current multidetector CT examinations with thinner collimations, generally cannot be characterized with confidence at CT. Because of the high prevalence of benign liver lesions, most of these are cysts, hemangiomas, biliary hamartomas, focal nodular hyperplasia, or hepatocellular adenomas. There is no guarantee of this, however, and it is incumbent on the imaging study properly to characterize these lesions. At CT, dis-

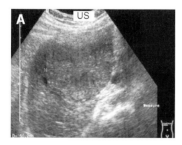 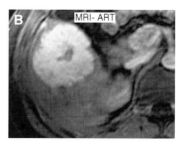 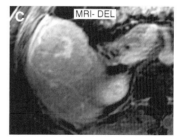

Fig. 7. A large FNH: US versus MR imaging. (*A*) US of the liver shows a large lesion with similar echogenicity as the surrounding liver. Subsequent MR imaging shows a classical FNH. (*B*) Gadolinium-enhanced MR imaging in the arterial phase shows intense homogenous enhancement of the entire lesion except the central scar and the septae. (*C*) In the delayed phase, the central scar and the septae are enhanced.

tinction between a small benign liver lesion and a metastasis or small HCC can be difficult (Fig. 8). The major strength of multidetector CT is the ability to show the hepatic vascular (mainly arterial) anatomy. This, however, does not facilitate better characterization of focal or diffuse liver lesions.

MR imaging provides a more comprehensive work-up of focal and diffuse liver disease. This is based on the unique properties of MR imaging that possess a combination of high intrinsic soft tissue contrast of the liver and liver lesions; various distinctly different tissue characteristics that are imaged; high sensitivity for the presence or absence of intravenous nonspecific contrast (gadolinium); and liver-specific contrast media. Because MR imaging lacks the hazards of ionizing radiation, most centers perform a multiphasic gadolinium-enhanced examination as a standard part of their work-up of liver diseases. Unlike CT, many centers have been routinely using a dynamic multiphasic (often three or more phases) gadolinium-enhanced imaging protocol as the standard MR imaging investigation in patients with suspected liver disease for more than a decade [10,11,25]. Dynamic gadolinium-enhanced imaging is considered essential in detection and characterization of liver lesions. For most body MR imaging radiologists the enhancement patterns of various focal liver lesions (and their signal intensity characteristics on T2- and T1-weighted sequences) are well known for many years.

Some centers use specific MR imaging contrast media, such as superparamagnetic iron-oxide [21,26] and manganese [27], to detect focal liver lesions. There are several disadvantages related to this approach and to the use of specific contrast media. (1) Superparamagnetic iron-oxide is a T2* shortening agent and relies on T2-weighted images, which general contain more artifacts and less intrinsic signal than T1-weighted MR images. (2) Superparamagnetic iron-oxide and manganese contrast media often require two separate imaging sessions before and after injection of contrast media. This is related to the lengthier tissue uptake time of many of these contrast media. Two separate MR imaging examinations are more costly and cumbersome. (3) Specific contrast media (unless it is a combined perfusional-tissue specific agent) do not provide information concerning the vascularity of liver lesions, which is extremely important information that is routinely provided with gadolinium. (4) Many specific contrast media have more side effects than gadolinium both recognized and theoretical. A recent paper reported on the risk of manganese neurotoxicity (causing a Parkinson-like progressive extrapyramidal disorder) from increased systemic manganese. Manganese-DPDP releases free manganese into blood and tissues, where it is quickly bound or retained by tissues. The brain is the major target organ for manganese toxicity, in part because it retains manganese much longer than other tissues. Following chronic overexposure, manganese can produce a progressive, permanent neurodegenerative disorder, with few options for treatment and no cure. Although it remains unclear whether a single dose of Manganese-DPDP leads to any neurologic consequences, care should be taken to avoid repeated exposure to manganese [28].

Currently, newer contrast media (gadolinium-based, T1 shortening agents) are available that have dual, nonspecific (perfusional), and specific functionality with biliary excretion. The specific enhancement properties may be useful to distinguish between primary and secondary liver lesions and to visualize

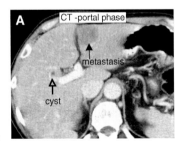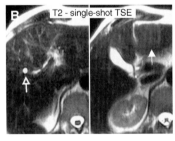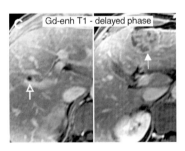

Fig. 8. Liver cyst versus liver metastasis. (*A*) Contrast-enhanced CT in the portal phase shows a small cyst (*open arrow*) that appears somewhat similar to the larger metastasis (*solid arrow*). (*B*) At T2-weighted single-shot turbo spin-echo (TSE) with a long echo time (120 milliseconds), the cyst is much brighter because of the high fluid content (*open arrow*), whereas the metastasis (*solid arrow*) is hardly visible indicating its solid nature. (*C*) Gadolinium-enhanced three-dimensional T1-weighted image in the delayed phase shows no enhancement of the cyst (*open arrow*), whereas the metastasis (*solid arrow*) shows typical heterogeneous enhancement. Based on the CT findings, a surgical decision was not possible, whereas based on the MR imaging findings, the patient confidently underwent a curative resection of the segments II and III.

the biliary tree. Compared with iodine-based contrast media used with CT, gadolinium-based MR imaging contrast media have several advantages. (1) T1-weighted MR imaging sequences are more sensitive to gadolinium than CT to iodine contrast media. This means that a smaller volume of MR imaging contrast (15–30 mL) can be used compared with the volume (150–200 mL) of iodine agents used for CT. (2) The viscosity of many of the gadolinium-based contrast media is lower than most iodine contrast media,

which can be important if high injection rates (> 4 mL/s) are required, for instance CT angiography with multidetector CT or MRA with parallel imaging. Because of the high viscosity of the iodine contrast media, insertion of larger-diameter needles is required for high injection rates for cardiac and vascular CT. This increases the complication rate at the site of injection including increased pain, increased number of needle sticks, increased size of local hematoma, and increased likelihood of subcutaneous injection of con-

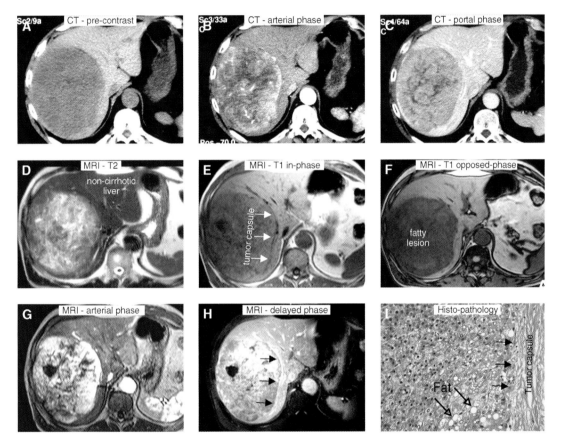

Fig. 9. Large liver tumor: CT versus MR imaging. A 41-year-old man without any history or evidence of liver disease presented with an incidental large liver tumor. (*A*) Unenhanced CT shows a hypodense tumor in the right lobe. (*B*) CT in the arterial phase shows enhancement of the tumor. (*C*) CT in the portal phase and delayed phase (not shown) shows washout in some areas. Based on CT, the exact nature of the lesion was not clear (the differential included hypervascular primary [adenoma, HCC] and secondary tumors [metastases]). MR imaging was performed. MR imaging shows no evidence of liver parenchymal disease (ie, no cirrhosis: normal signal on all sequences, smooth edges, no nodules). (*D*) On T2-weighted images the tumor was predominantly higher signal than liver. Chemical shift imaging (in-phase [*E*] and opposed-phase [*F*]) clearly shows evidence of fat within the tumor (note the decreased signal in the tumor on the opposed-phase image [*F*]). In addition, a low-intensity tumor capsule (*arrows*) is visible on the in-phase image (*E*). (*G*) On the gadolinium-enhanced MR imaging in the arterial phase the tumor shows intense heterogeneous enhancement with intratumoral vessels. (*H*) In the delayed phase, the tumor shows washout with enhancement of a tumor capsule (*arrows*). Based on the MR imaging findings of a large fat-containing hypervascular heterogeneous tumor with a tumor capsule, the diagnosis of a fatty HCC in a noncirrhotic liver was made and the patient underwent a curative resection. (*I*) At histopathology MR imaging findings were confirmed: a fat-containing (*open arrows*) HCC was surrounded by a true fibrous tumor capsule (*solid arrows*).

trast. Subcutaneous injection of the large volume of contrast at the high injection rates of CT can be a major health and litigation issue. (3) Gadolinium-based contrast media at clinically recommended doses are not nephrotoxic and can be injected even in the presence of renal insufficiency, which is not true for CT.

Because CT mainly relies on the vascularity of liver lesions, and lacks the ability to alter intrinsic soft tissue contrast, as MR imaging is able to do (eg, with variable T1- and T2-weighting, selective fat-suppression, chemical shift, and diffusion weighting), not only small (< 2 cm) but also larger lesions may be difficult to characterize at CT (Fig. 9). This is particularly true with the incidental finding of a single hypervascular lesion without any history of parenchymal liver disease or any underlying malignancy.

In such cases, MR imaging can provide essential and very specific tissue characteristics of the lesion and the surrounding liver (cirrhosis versus noncirrhosis) and hence can considerably narrow down the differential to only one or two entities or even provide a very specific diagnosis (Fig. 10). More importantly, state-of-the-art MR imaging facilitates clinical and surgical decision-making with confidence in most patients with inconclusive US and CT examinations.

For many primary hypervascular liver lesions, like focal nodular hyperplasia, hepatocellular adenoma, most small hemangiomas, HCC, and some hypervascular metastases, such as melanoma metastases (Fig. 11), FDG-PET is false-negative. In the authors' experience, the accuracy of state-of-the-art MR imaging is unparalleled in such entities. At this point

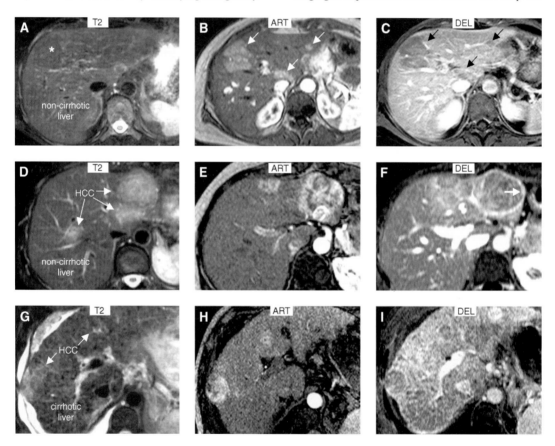

Fig. 10. Multiple adenomas versus multiple HCC. (A–C) Multiple adenomas. The largest of the three adenomas (*) is slightly hypointense on this fat-suppressed T2-weighted sequence because of high fatty content of the lesion (A). The other two lesions are isointense and the liver is noncirrhotic (smooth edges, no atrophy or hypertrophy of segments, no nodules). In the arterial phase (B), the three adenomas (arrows) show homogeneous blush of enhancement. In the delayed phase (C), the lesions show no heterogeneity or tumor capsule (arrows). (D–F) Multiple HCC in a noncirrhotic liver. HCCs are brighter than the liver with intense heterogeneous enhancement, washout, and enhancing tumor capsule (arrow in F). (G–I) Multiple HCC in a cirrhotic liver. The cirrhotic liver contains numerous regenerative dark nodules and two brighter larger lesions with characteristics of HCC (mildly hyperintense on T2 with enhancement, washout, and enhanced tumor capsule).

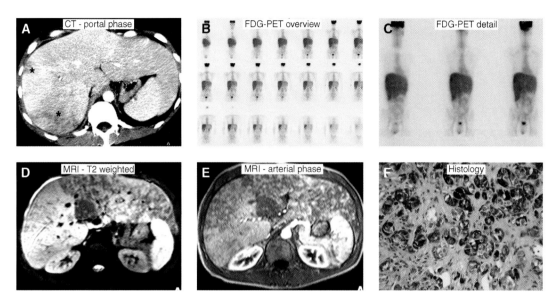

Fig. 11. Melanoma liver metastases: comparison of CT, FDG-PET, and MR imaging. A 36-year-old man with a history of melanoma developed abnormal liver function tests and underwent a single-phase CT (*A*), which showed two large abnormalities in the right liver (*). (*B,C*) A FDG-PET, performed within 2 weeks after CT, showed no abnormalities. In particular, the liver was considered to have normal activity. Subsequently, MR imaging of the liver (1 week after PET) revealed diffuse focal lesions. The signal intensity and the enhancement were compatible with diffuse melanoma metastases. T1-weighted images (not shown) demonstrated high signal abnormal patchy areas (because of the presence of melanin). T2-weighted image (*D*) showed diffuse and patchy increased signal intensity, and gadolinium-enhanced T1-weighted image in the arterial phase (*E*) showed diffuse and patchy enhancement of the lesions. Because of the confusing results of the different imaging modalities, an US-guided biopsy was performed of lesions in the right and left lobe. Microphotograph (hematoxylin and eosin, original magnification ×200) showed diffuse sinusoidal infiltration of the liver with melanin-containing (dark) cells (*F*) and hence confirmed the findings of MR imaging (see Fig. 4M–O).

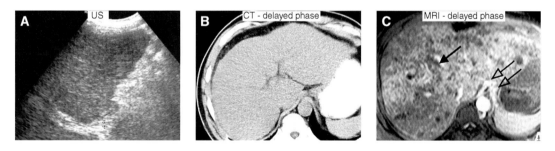

Fig. 12. A 44-year-old man with liver disease presented with variceal bleeding and increased levels of alfa fetoprotein: US, CT, and MR imaging findings. (*A*) US of the liver shows a diffuse echogenic liver. No tumor or cause of the bleeding was seen. (*B*) A following CT (1 day after US) showed no distinct abnormalities or cause of the bleeding. At other levels, areas with vascular abnormalities were described at CT (not shown). Gadolinium-enhanced MR imaging (1 day after CT) demonstrated heterogeneous enhancement of the entire liver with patchy areas of washout in a typical cirrhotic liver (irregular margins, hypertrophy of segment I, slight hypertrophy of the right liver). (*C*) Note also the portal vein with enhanced tumor thrombosis (*solid arrow*). The findings on T2-weighted with patchy increased signal (not shown) and gadolinium-enhanced images were compatible with diffuse HCC with portal invasion. MR imaging also showed ascites and large esophageal varices (*open arrows*), which caused the bleeding.

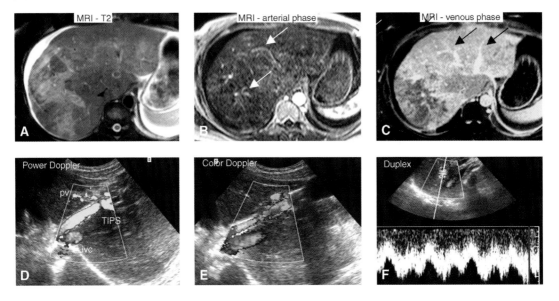

Fig. 13. Budd-Chiari syndrome. Diagnosis (MR imaging) (*A–C*) and transjugular intrahepatic portosystemic shunt (TIPS) evaluation (US) (*D–F*). T2-weighted MR imaging shows abnormal high signal in the periphery of the liver (*), whereas the central part (segment I) is enlarged with normal low signal (*A*). Gadolinium-enhanced MR imaging in the arterial (*B*) and delayed (*C*) phases show intrahepatic collaterals (*arrows*). Power Doppler (*D*), color Doppler (*E*), and duplex (*F*) can be used for evaluation of the blood flow in TIPS.

in time, FDG-PET is not suitable for clinical or surgical decision-making in patients with suspected primary liver lesions or melanoma metastases. The greatest strength of FDG-PET compared with all other imaging modalities is the staging of lung cancers [29].

Diffuse liver abnormalities

These include a number metabolic, depositional, vascular, and biliary tree abnormalities. Important examples are focal or diffuse fatty infiltration of the

liver; hereditary hemochromatosis; iron deposition disease (hemosiderosis); chronic liver disease; cirrhosis; Budd-Chiari syndrome; Caroli's disease; and primary sclerosing cholangitis. Diffuse malignant disease can be considered in this category because it must be distinguished from benign disease; a prime example is diffuse HCC [7]. All these disease entities can be diagnosed with high accuracy at state-of-the-art MR imaging (Figs. 12–15). Other modalities, such as US and CT, are often inconclusive for diffuse liver abnormalities. MR imaging should be the modality of choice for all suspected or known diffuse

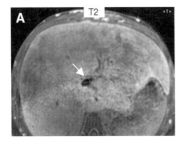
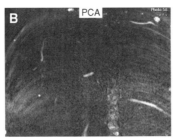
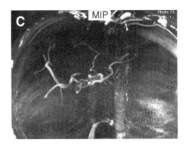

Fig. 14. Budd-Chiari syndrome. TIPS evaluation with phase-contrast MRA (PCA). Because of the large size of the liver, US did not allow the visualization of the TIPS (not shown). A contrast-enhanced CT was inconclusive (not shown). (*A*) A T2-weighted MR image shows the TIPS as signal void (*arrow*). (*B*) A phase-contrast MRA (velocity encoding 15 cm/s) showed signal in the intrahepatic collaterals but no signal in the TIPS and the inferior vena cava, compatible with thrombosis of both vessels. (*C*) A MIP of the PCA provides an overview of the intrahepatic and abdominal wall collaterals.

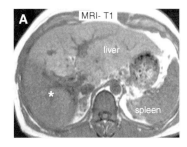 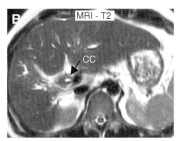 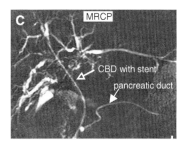

Fig. 15. Primary sclerosing cholangitis complicated with a cholangiocarcinoma. A patient with known primary sclerosing cholangitis developed a sudden increase in cholestatic liver function tests and underwent an endoscopic retrograde cholangiopancreatography with stenting of the common bile duct, and subsequently MR imaging and MR cholangiopancreatography. Endoscopic retrograde cholangiopancreatography was inconclusive for malignancy. (*A*) T1-weighted MR image shows abnormal low signal intensity in most of the right part of the liver. (*B*) T2-weighted MR imaging (single-shot, heavily T2-weighted sequence) shows a localized common bile duct wall thickening (>3 mm), which caused a dominant stenosis compatible with cholangiocarcinoma. (*C*) MR cholangiopancreatography provides an overview of the intrahepatic bile ducts with variable dilatations and narrowing, which is typical for primary sclerosing cholangitis. Note the common bile duct with a stent and the normal aspect of the pancreatic duct. CBD, common bile duct; CC, cholangiocarcinoma.

liver abnormalities. For the assessment of vascular structures, US with color or power Doppler may also be used. If the liver increases in size or in the presence of ascites, however, it may be technically difficult to assess flow with US. In such cases, phase-contrast MRA may be used to assess and even quantify flow (see Figs. 13 and 14).

Hepatic imaging: systematic review of the literature

To perform a thorough systematic review of the relevant literature, a MEDLINE search of the English-language literature was performed to identify original articles describing the imaging of focal liver lesions between 1980 and 2004. Combinations of the following search terms were used:

Ultrasound (US)
Computed tomography (CT)
Computed tomography
    arterioportography (CTAP)
MR imaging (MRI)
Positron emission tomography (PET)
Diagnosis
Liver
Liver lesions
Metastasis
Hepatocellular carcinoma
Hepatocellular adenoma
Focal nodular hyperplasia

In addition, the reference lists of the individual papers found by MEDLINE search and national and international experts in abdominal imaging were consulted to provide suggestions for the relevant literature. Review papers and papers concerning meta-analysis were excluded. The articles were selected for analysis based on the following criteria: (1) the article was in the English language; (2) the standard of reference was defined in the paper; (3) imaging modality was used as part of the preoperative work-up; and (4) the article provided specific information on one or more of the following statistical measures: sensitivity, specificity, positive predictive value, negative predictive value, accuracy, area under the receiver operating characteristic (ROC) curve, or the absolute number of true-positives, true-negatives, false-positives, and false-negatives.

Consolidating the information provided in the systematic review of the current literature shows that MR imaging of the liver is the best modality for preoperative imaging of focal liver lesions. The area under the ROC curve (Az) values of MR imaging are 0.90 or higher in most studies, whereas those of CT and CTAP are below 0.90 [11,12,21,22,30,31]. These findings are summarized in a scatterplot of the true-positive rate versus false-positive rates of US, CT, CTAP, MR imaging, and PET (Fig. 16). Formal quantitative pooling of sensitivities and specificities or summary ROC analysis was not possible primarily because many studies lacked information on the number of true-negative diagnoses. This is to be expected in the clinical setting, because benign lesions are often not confirmed by biopsy or controlled follow-up.

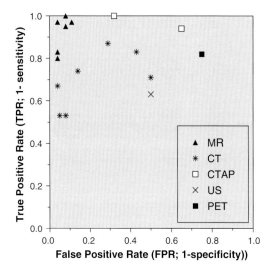

Fig. 16. Hepatic imaging: a graph compares the false-positive and the true-positive rates of US, CT, CT arteriography, MR imaging, and PET. The data for the graph are obtained from a systematic review of the literature. CTAP, CT arteriography.

The sensitivity of MR imaging is between 80% and 100% for focal liver lesions, that of CT 53% to 87%, and that of CTAP 70% to 96%. The specificity of MR imaging and CT was comparable (up to 96%), whereas CTAP had a much lower specificity (around 80%) mainly resulting from false-positive findings caused by pseudolesions and the presence of benign lesions (Table 2) [3,4,11–14,20,26,31–35].

PET is a newer imaging technique that is currently less available than US, CT, and MR imaging. There are a few comparative studies for the detection and characterization of focal liver lesions. A recent comparative study concluded that the sensitivity and specificity of PET (82% and 25%, respectively) for the detection of primary and secondary liver lesions was superior to US (63% and 50%) and CT (71% and 50%) but not to MR imaging (83% and 57%, respectively) [33]. PET has limited spatial resolution compared with CT and MR imaging, and the intrinsic heterogeneous activity in normal background liver further limits the ability of FDG-PET to show small malignant lesions. This is further compounded by the unpredictably variable FDG uptake, in all cases of malignant lesions, but especially in the postchemotherapy setting PET will most likely play a role in

Table 2
Imaging modalities and liver lesions: sensitivity, specificity, and positive and negative predictive values

First author, year [Ref.]	Lesions		Modality	Sn (%)	Sp (%)	PPV (%)	NPV (%)
	N	Type					
McFarland, 1994 [11]	82	Benign and malignant	MR imaging	100	92	—	—
Soyer, 1996 [14]	108	Benign and malignant	MR imaging	83	—	—	—
Semelka, 1999 [20]	85	Metastases	**MR imaging**-CTAP[a]	96, 87	97, 71	98, 90	92, 65
Ward, 1999 [31]	197	Benign and metastases	CT	75	—	—	—
			SPIO-MR imaging	80	—	—	—
Jang, 2000 [34]	73	HCC	**CT**-CTAP- CTHA[a]	94, 96, 97	—	96, 65, 80	—
Bluemke, 2000 [26]	82	Metastases	**CT**-MR imaging[a]	67, 80	96, 96	—	—
Schmidt, 2000 [13]	33	Metastases	**Helical CT**-CTAP[a]	53, 100	92, 68	—	—
Reimer, 2000 [21]	35	Benign and malignant	**CT**-SPIO-MR imaging[a]	74, 97	86, 89	—	—
Kim, 2001 [32]	86	Small hemangiomas and hypervascular metastases	Triphasic CT	53	95	—	—
Haider, 2002 [3]	88	Benign and metastases	CT	82	—	—	—
Coulam, 2002 [4]	114	TND	MR imaging	83	96	100	—
Laghi, 2003 [35]	140	HCC	CT	87	—	94	—
Bohm, 2004 [33]	174	TND	**PET**-US-CT-MR imaging[a]	82, 63, 71, 83	25, 50, 50, 57	96, 96, 97, 97	—

Abbreviations: NPV, negative predictive value; PPV, positive predictive value, Sn, sensitivity; Sp, specificity; TND, type not defined.
    [a] Comparative study. Values relate to modality in boldface.

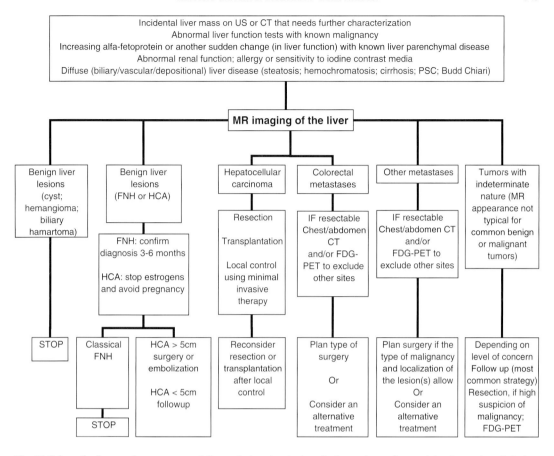

Fig. 17. Schematic diagram shows a proposed diagnostic imaging strategy for the work-up of suspected or known hepatic lesion. HCA, hepatocellular adenoma.

staging and particularly exclusion of extrahepatic disease in the future, and the future impact of new PET tracers.

Summary: proposed strategy for comprehensive hepatic imaging

A large number of comparative studies concerning the preoperative imaging of focal liver lesions have been published. Many studies have various limitations. Nevertheless, a number of conclusions can be drawn: MR imaging has a larger area under the ROC curve than US, CT, and CTAP. MR imaging has a higher sensitivity and specificity than US, CT, CTAP, or PET. The findings from the literature suggest that the state-of-the-art MR imaging of the liver should play a pivotal role as a comprehensive approach for the work-up of patients with suspected or known liver abnormalities (Fig. 17). Modern CT is the most comparable modality to MR imaging in its overall

diagnostic accuracy, but a use of MR imaging will be the increasing concern of the risks of cancer induction by excessive use of CT.

Acknowledgments

The authors are grateful to Myriam G.M. Hunink, MD (Professor of Radiology and Epidemiology), for advice concerning the systematic review of the literature, and Linda Everse (Research Coordinator) for assistance with the preparation of the tables and graphs of the systematic review.

References

[1] Karhunen PJ. Benign hepatic tumours and tumour-like conditions in men. J Clin Pathol 1986;39:183–8.
[2] Schwartz LH, Gandras EJ, Colangelo SM, et al. Prevalence and importance of small hepatic lesions

found at CT in patients with cancer. Radiology 1999; 210:71–4.

[3] Haider MA, Amital MM, Rappaport DC, et al. Multi-detector row helical CT in preoperative assessment of small (≤1.5 cm) liver metastases: is thinner collimation better? Radiology 2002;225:137–42.

[4] Coulam CH, Chan FP, Li KC. Can a multiphasic contrast-enhanced three-dimensional fast spoiled gradient-recalled echo sequence be sufficient for liver MR imaging? AJR Am J Roentgenol 2002;178:335–41.

[5] Valls C, Andia E, Sanchez A, et al. Hepatic metastases from colorectal cancer: preoperative detection and assessment of resectability with helical CT. Radiology 2001;218:55–60.

[6] Yoon SS, Tanabe TK. Surgical treatment and other regional treatments for colorectal cancer liver metastases. Oncologist 1999;4:197–208.

[7] Hussain SM, Semelka RC, Mitchell DG. MR imaging of hepatocellular carcinoma. Magn Reson Imaging Clin N Am 2002;10:31–52.

[8] Hussain SM, Zondervan PE, Ijzermans JN, et al. Benign versus malignant hepatic nodules: MR imaging findings with pathologic correlation. Radiographics 2002;22:1023–36.

[9] Semelka RC, Hussain SM, Marcos HB, et al. Biliary hamartomas on MRI: common entity, rarely diagnosed. J Magn Reson Imaging 1999;10:196–201.

[10] McFarland EG, Mayo-Smith WW, Saini S, et al. Hepatic hemangiomas and malignant tumors: improved differentiation with heavily T2-weighted conventional spin-echo MR imaging. Radiology 1994; 193:43–7.

[11] Mitchell DG, Saini S, Weinreb J, et al. Hepatic metastases and cavernous hemangiomas: distinction with standard- and triple-dose gadoteridol-enhanced MR imaging. Radiology 1994;193:49–57.

[12] Terkivatan T, Hussain SM, Lameris JS, et al. Transcatheter arterial embolization as a safe and effective treatment for focal nodular hyperplasia of the liver. Cardiovasc Intervent Radiol 2002;25:450–3.

[13] Schmidt J, Strotzer M, Fraunhofer S, et al. Intraoperative ultrasonography versus helical computed tomography and computed tomography with arterioportography in diagnosing colorectal liver metastases: lesion-by-lesion analysis. World J Surg 2000;24:43–8.

[14] Soyer P, de Givry SC, Gueye C, et al. Detection of focal hepatic lesions with MR imaging: prospective comparison of T2-weighted fast spin-echo with and without fat suppression, T2-weighted breath-hold fast spin-echo, and gadolinium chelate-enhanced 3D gradient-recalled imaging. AJR Am J Roentgenol 1996;166:1115–21.

[15] de Rave S, Hussain SM. A liver tumour as an incidental finding: differential diagnosis and treatment. Scand J Gastroenterol Suppl 2002;236:81–6.

[16] Bryant T, Blomley M, Albrecht T, et al. Improved characterization of liver lesions with liver-phase uptake of liver-specific microbubbles: prospective multicenter study. Radiology 2004;232:799–809.

[17] Entrekin RR, Porter BA, Sillesen HH, et al. Real-time spatial compound imaging: application to breast, vascular, and musculoskeletal ultrasound. Semin Ultrasound CT MR 2001;22:50–64.

[18] Flanagan FL, Dehdashti F, Ogunbiyi OA, et al. Utility of FDG-PET for investigating unexplained plasma CEA elevation in patients with colorectal cancer. Ann Surg 1998;227:319–23.

[19] Hussain SM, De Becker J, Hop WCJ, et al. Can a single-shot black-blood T2-weighted spin-echo echo planar imaging sequence with sensitivity encoding replace the respiratory-triggered turbo spin-echo sequence for the liver? An optimization and a feasibility study. J Magn Reson Imaging 2005;21:219–29.

[20] Semelka RC, Cance WG, Marcos HB, et al. Liver metastases: comparison of current MR techniques and spiral CT during arterial portography for detection in 20 surgically staged cases. Radiology 1999;213: 86–91.

[21] Reimer P, Jahnke N, Fiebich M, et al. Hepatic lesion detection and characterization: value of nonenhanced MR imaging. Superparamagnetic iron oxide-enhanced MR imaging, and spiral CT: ROC analysis. Radiology 2000;217:152–8.

[22] Seneterre E, Taorel P, Bouvier Y, et al. Detection of hepatic metastases: ferumoxides-enhanced MR imaging versus unenhanced MR imaging and CT during arterio-portography. Radiology 1996;200:785–92.

[23] Wang YX, Hussain SM, Krestin GP. Superparamagnetic iron oxide contrast media: physicochemical characteristics and applications in MR imaging. Eur Radiol 2001;11:19–31.

[24] Hussain SM, Terkivatan T, Zondervan PE, et al. Focal nodular hyperplasia: findings at state-of-the-art MR imaging, ultrasound, CT and pathologic analysis. Radiographics 2004;24:3–19.

[25] Outwater E, Tomaszewski JE, Daly JM, et al. Hepatic colorectal metastases: correlation of MR imaging and pathologic appearance. Radiology 1991;180:327 32.

[26] Bluemke DA, Paulson EK, Choti MA, et al. Detection of hepatic lesions in candidates for surgery: comparison of ferumoxides-enhanced MR imaging and dual-phase helical CT. AJR Am J Roentgenol 2000;175: 1653–8.

[27] Braga HJV, Choti MA, Lee VS, et al. Liver lesion: manganese-enhanced MR and dual-phase helical CT for preoperative detection and characterization. Comparison with receiver operating characteristic analysis. Radiology 2002;223:525–31.

[28] Crossgrove J, Zheng W. Manganese toxicity upon over exposure. NMR Biomed 2004;17:544–53.

[29] Antoch G, Vogt FM, Freudenberg LS, et al. Whole-body dual-modality PET/CT and whole-body MRI for tumor staging in oncology. JAMA 2003;290: 3199–206.

[30] Pauleit D, Textor J, Bachmann R, et al. Hepatocellular carcinoma: detection with gadolinium- and ferumoxides-enhanced MR imaging of the liver. Radiology 2002;222:73–80.

[31] Ward J, Naik KS, Guthrie IA, et al. Comparison of MR imaging after the administration of superparamagnetic iron oxide with dual-phase CT by using alternative-free response operating characteristic analysis. Radiology 1999;210:459–66.

[32] Kim T, Federle MP, Baron RL, et al. Discrimination of small hepatic hemangiomas from hypervascular malignant tumors smaller than 3 cm with three-phase helical CT. Radiology 2001;219:699–706.

[33] Bohm B, Voth M, Geoghegan J, et al. Impact of PET on strategy in liver resection for primary and secondary liver tumors. J Cancer Res Clin Oncol 2004; 130:266–72.

[34] Jang H-J, Lim JH, Lee SJ, et al. Hepatocellular carcinoma: are combined CT during arterial portography and CT hepatic arteriography in addition to triple-phase helical CT all necessary for preoperative evaluation? Radiology 2000;215:373–80.

[35] Laghi A, Iannaccone R, Rossi P, et al. Hepatocellular carcinoma: detection with triple-phase multidetector row helical CT in patients with chronic hepatitis. Radiology 2003;226:543–9.

ELSEVIER
SAUNDERS

Radiol Clin N Am 43 (2005) 949–952

RADIOLOGIC
CLINICS
of North America

Index

Note: Page numbers of article titles are in **boldface** type.